A   LITTLE WAY TO YOGA

A SIMPLE WAY TO PRACTICE YOGA

NARRATED BY

DR.S.JAYA KUMAR

PREFACE

The mind power of a human beings can bring everything in front of his eyes ,if it is used in a proper way, Among the living beings in the earth human is differentiated by his mind power .some person used this mind as a friend but in other person in act negatively .All the problem in the life are created by the non understanding the matter ,even though there is proper development of body and brain .

So proper controlling of the mind is necessary for all human beings ,it only brings happiness to us .the yoga is gifted to the world by the ancient tradition of India ,the ultimate divine power of YOGA is unite every living beings in the earth by love .

In modern days the world is restlessness ,all activity are based on money earning only ,so, competition is inevitable in the world. It creates some rival jealousy among the country level, among the society level, and among the family level it will reflected. The divine power for YOGA will give enthusiasm and energetic ,bring happiness to the follower .for this reason the yoga is practiced through the age, by the ancient sages of India .

Many people come from across various part of the world whenever we meet, we defiantly talk about the YOGA so I give many time literature about YOGA ,Many friends of various country asking me to publish a book about yoga and postural exercise. show I decide THAT MY WORK WILL DIFFER FROM OTHER BOOKS ,as a ayurvedic physician here I will correlate ayurveda with yoga science and give this book to you. As a AYURVWEDIC physician I have give solution for many diseases and disorder by the YOGA SCIENCE .

In eight fold of YOGA the ASANAM [postural]get very important roll .it can easily follow up ,and performed by the people living all over the world . This book come with a small introduction of our body in ayurvedic way .and introduction to yoga and postural performance ,do's and don'ts in yoga ,dress code ,food and dietic regimens also explained in this books, this will also very helpful to Our readers .this book is useful for all age group those who practice yoga or not .

In fourteen years of my teaching experience in ayurveda and yogic science ,

I carefully prepare this books as much give more concentration for this work ,dear reader as much as information is possible I given with proper reference ,so please come with me ,we have to travel sometime along with my text and, I have teach you about the immortal yoga science ......

BY

DR.S. JAYA KUMAR

COPY RIGHT DISCLAIMER

THIS TEXT IS BASED ON INDIAN LANGUAGE, FOR MEANING PLEASE USE THE ANNEXURE PAGE:

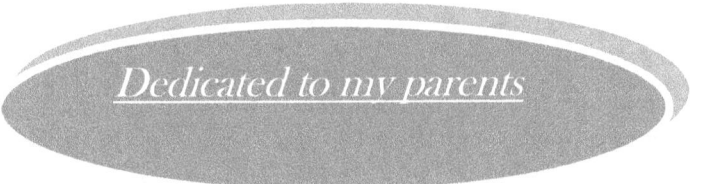

Dedicated to my parents

CONTENT

INTRODUCTION

YOGA IS A GIFT TO THE WORLD

Dear Readers , There are many more authors had described about the science of yoga especially, they more concentrate about the posture practices ,am not new one .The yoga science has developed more powerfully after the grant visit of swamy Vivekananda to the western country in yearly 19 century .The science of yoga has practiced more than two thousand years in India, but the speed of development is limited .The yoga has practiced by sages and saints of the India ,the practice of yoga by the citizen is limited later the period the citizen has to practiced the yoga science .

Various archaeological study and stone sculpture, provide strong evidence of the yoga how much it spread throughout the country ,various king and emperor have provide subsidy to various yoga schools conducted by saint and sages .In recent days there are many yoga schools has teaching to the various people ,in India and other country .the government of India has given more attention to development of yoga .

The UNO has announced international yoga day on June 21 of every year .in UNGA meeting held on twenty seven September 2015, Our honourable prime minister has proposed the significance yoga ,and it need of every people all over the world ,in that meeting he tell about yoga is a invaluable gift of India 's ancient tradition to the world .

On the strong recommendation and proposal of our prime minister in UNGA .India 's permanent representative ASHOK MUKHERJI has introduced the draft resolution in UNGA ,177memebers support without vote the resolution has passed in the UNGA .and UNO has announced the 21 st June of every year will celebrate the international yoga day.

Dear reader am not new one to give lecture about the yoga science ,there are many yoga schools are conducted by sages in India and foreign country , they are delivered lot of speech and print lot of manual ,its free to high level dollar s depend upon the popularity of the sages ,.

But my work is entirely different ,When I was sixteen ,I completed my higher secondary school, with lot of imagination ,and thoughts I planned for my college education ,after long struggle I have joined in under graduate AYURVEDA PHYSICIAN course .the seat allotted for me in under rural category ,in that day provisional government had allocated some seats for student who complete their study in village area .In that category ,I joined my under graduate degree in sriperumbudhur, kancheepuram district.

History of ayurveda is one of the main subject in1998 batch student ,in this chapter we discussed about the history of ayurveda how it originate ,how its spread ,in this chapter one word give more interesting to us ,that word is SIDDHAR that super natural people who lived Indian sub continent ,they well versed in various field example medicine ,astrology, architecture ,kayakalpam (immortal of life with medicine)philosophy etc.

Before going to practice the yoga and postural exercise, one must to know about his sareeram (BODY)how is our body is formed ,the relation between PANCHA MAHA BOOTHAM {WATER ,EARTH,FIRE ,ETHER ,AIR } and the body ,relation between dosas and dhathus ,relation between dhathus and waste product .etc ,you must know each and every thing before you going to entered to practice the postural exercise .In some mutt they going to taught only yoga and postural exercise ,but sometime the aggravation of dosas in the body will lead to destruct our body .

The dosas can able to perform to maintain the body function ,and they can able to destruct our body and lead to mortal ,one simple example is there when you going to study car driving the trainer first he explain the mechanism in the car ,function of the engine ,spark plug ,battery maintaining ,brake maintaining fluid level maintenance extra ,then only he give train us to drive the vehicle .

For attain above the super natural power the YOGA FOUNDATION IS ESSENTIAL, yoga not only for physical body as well as good mental balance has to be provided by the yoga,

So, My dear sisters and brothers today ,I have to illustrated about the science of yoga, which was different from other authors .because mostly all authors are yoga follower traditionally from master to student .

Am in the field of *medical science of ayurveda* nearly twenty years of experience and teaching field of yoga nearly fourteen years of experience . The three dosas theory is essential, to maintain good health apart from three dosas there are seven dhathus ,and three malas is there .these only the construct the good health to us they can able to maintain good health ,and they can able to destruct the body .

The three basic elements support to the mind and the body , they are

For mind controlling factor

1	SATTVAM
2	RAJAS
3	THAMAS

The three dosas

The body controlling factor

1 – VATA

2 - PITTAM

3 - KAPHAM

They constitute the body ,They have dominant in morning ,afternoon, evening .age wise young ,middle ,old ,

when these factors are predominant in at the time of intercourse the semen and ovum joined the zygote is produced ,they constitute the body so there are three individual constitution .

VATA PRAKRUTHI	-VATA
PITTA PRAKRUTHI	-PITTAM
KAPHA PRAKRUTHI	-KAPHAM

VATA PITTA PRAKRUTHI	VATA+PITTAM
VATA KAPHA PRAKRUTHI	-VATA+KAPHAM
PITTA KAPHA PRAKRUTHI	-PITTA+KAPHAM

SAMA PRAKRUTHI	-VATA+PITTA+KAPHAM

These are called as single prakruthis or constitution, and each two joined and produced prakruthis called as DWIDOSAJA.AND total three joined produced SANNIPATHJA PRAKRUTHI .Depend upon the constitution each person activity is different ,food acceptance also different ,this may affect the person in climate changes .

The three basic dosas are constituted by **PANCHA MAHA BOOTHAM**, each **DOSHA** there is involvement of the panchamahabootham are five elements;

PRITHVI	-EARTH
AP	-WATER
THEJAS	-FIRE
VAYU	-AIR
AKASAM	-ETHER

Relation between five elements and body

VATA	-VAYU	-AKASAM-ETHER
PITTAM	-FIRE	-WATER+FIRE
KAPHAM	-EARTH	-WATER+EARTH

Out of from these there are seven basic tissues are present in our body.

RASAM –PLASMA---WATER

RAKTHAM—BLOOD---FIRE+WATER

MAMASAM—WATER---PRITHVI

MEDAS— LIPIDS---PRITHVI+WATER

ASTHI—BONE---PRITHVI+AKASAM

MAJJA—MARROW---WATER+VAYU

SUKRAM—SEMAN---WATER+PRITHVI

THERE ARE THREE WASTE PRODUCT IN OUR BODY.

1- PURISHA   FEACES   - EARTH+AIR

2- MUTRA   URINE   -WATER+FIRE

3- SWETA   SWEATING   -WATER+VAYU

So before going to practice the yoga and postural exercise, one must to know about his sareeram BODY how is our body is formed ,the relation between panchamahabootham and the body ,relation between dosha and dhathus ,relation between dhathus and waste product .etc SO ,here I explain the some part of the AYURVEDA for knowing purpose only.

Dear reader, The origin of yoga is differ from text to text .In SINDHU RIVER VALLY period has provide some valuable information about yoga science has practiced in those days .the broken earthen pots symbols, and meditation symbols of lord PASUPATHY and black drawing diagram, Has provide the evidence of yoga has practiced in *HARAPPA AND MAHANJADHARO* period also .The time period of sindhu river valley is more than three thousand seven fifty years old. By confirmed various carbon study conducted by archaeologist.

In rig Vedic verses the word yoga is founded ,the rig VEDA is mainly perform for Vedic ritual in the form of poem .There are nearly one thousand and one hundred fifty poem is founded .the lord worshiped in the name of agni (fire), and it was oldest more than five thousand years old .Apart from this in *MAHABHARATHA lord KRISHNA DELEVERD THE GREAT BAGAVAT GITHA* ,which was old nearly 500bce .In BAGAVAT GITHA the lord give seventeen chapter related to various philosophy ,He mainly described about KARMA YOGA and BAKTHI YOGAM concept .

The later the great sage *PATHANJALI* only described about the yoga in eight fold method is called as *ASTANGA YOGA* .the origin of sage PATHANJALI is in the form of *ADHI SESAN* is snake bed, used by LORD VISHNU ,.There is one mythological study has deals about his origin in the earth .

One day the snake god he feel heavy weight as compare with normal weight of lord Vishnu, so he ask this difference to lord .Then lord replied he was seen the GREAT COSMIC DANCE OF LORD SIVA so I was very happy that time .so, my weight is increased ,THEN the SERPENT ADHISESAN want to see the cosmic dance so, he tell his wish to lord VISNU .he advised to take birth in CHIDAMPARAM ,SO ,the snack come to earth and take the origin and get PATHANJALLI name .

Due to his divine nature with powerful poison he never seen anybody .When his breath is fall on somebody ,they become in to ash .whenever he going to take lesson to his student ,there is screen in front of him .One day he teach to his student ,one of the interesting disciples removed the screen .the thousand students of PATHANJALLI become to ashes .only one guy was escaped due to he went another place for other work dictated by the sages. the disciples is called as KANAPATHR ,.SO the sage feel very sad about this incident and he taught all lesson to that particular student .

There are many person described about yoga ,but ,lord PATHANJALLI only give good explanation about the yoga .he tell ....

//: YUJI YATHE ITHI YOGAHA //:

The above verses is give the etymology of the word yoga ,the route word of is come from *yuj* this meaning is to UNITE or joint ,to joint our internal soul to external soul of cosmic, is the main aim of the yoga .

//: YOGAHA SIDHA VRITHI NIRODHAHA //

In the above verses, he give the definition about yoga., The main function of the yoga is to prevent our increase of thinking .when a person try to control his mind is not possible in initial stage so our mind compared to a **MONKEY** ,it is not stable in one place ,it will jump one tree to other tree ,it will disturb other animal by catching the tail and legs ,even the great lion and tiger also suffered by monkey .like that our mind will be acted .so ,the yoga will help to us and concentrate our mind to focus one point .and help to us to attain the salvation.

For controlling the mind in initial stage it can't possible ,so, step by step only our mind will come our control ,for this goal Sage pathanjali give demonstrate EIGHT FOLD OF YOGA like following,

YAMA

NIYAMA

ASANAM

PRANAYAMAM

PRATHYAKARAM

DHARANAM

DHYANAM

SAMADHI

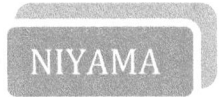

The etymology of the word YAMA means attitude towards our living situation ,these include five subtypes *,NON VIOLENCE,NOT TELLING LYING,NOT STEALING,CELEBACY,NON POSSESSIVNESS* ,these are the five qualities are involved in the YAMA.A yogi should follow this in initial step then he will get discipline in body and mind this will reflect his daily character .

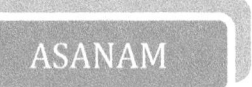

 It is the second anga of the ASTANGA YOGA ,this part mainly deals with how a person to take care about the body ,he should always maintain PURITY,HAPPINESS,DEVTION TO GOD,SEKF STUDY {TO ANALYSIS THE GOOD AND BAD activity done by him to others} YAGNA performs in front of fire god.

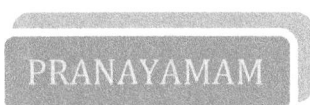

THE COMFORTABLE SITING POSTURE is called as POSTURE or asanam ,in this book we have elaborately to study this part ,so dear reader this much definition is enough.

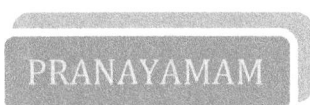

The etymology of the word PRANAYAMA means breathing exercise ,in the MOOLADHARAM the KUNDALI power is sleep like a serpent, the two NADI is originated in the MOOLADHARAM and travel in a crisscross manner and reach the brain

,during the this travel they met in SIX place ,SO , total along with MOOLADHARAM is six in number ,it called SAD CHAKRAS ,IT IS THE NORMAL PHYSIOLOICAL FUNCTION IS ROUTINE IN DAILY LIFE ,But when doing BREATHING exercise the sleeping KUNDALI IS WAKEUP and reach the brain and produced the nectar .so the YOGI live long without any food ,but the kundali in every AADHARAM it will show some effects ,so proper guidance is essential.

PRATHYAKARA

The etymology of the word PRATHYAKARAM means give stir our senses to contact the external thing .control our thinking is essential for YOGIS ,because the every contact with external object our mind lead to increase imagination power, so mind control is essential for yogi ,this PRATHYAKARAM help to him to prevent such things.

DHARANAM

Is the initial step to deep meditation ,the etymology of the word DHARANAM means to holding our sense and focused in a particular point ,.when doing this our meditation power will get improved .

DHYANAM

In recent days the word DHYANAM is very popular even though children also they perform the dhyanam .the etymology of the word DHYANAM means meditation ,it is the next step to DHARANAM ,the focused mind has develop to perform the meditation .but now a days without proper training some people perform the meditation which will lead to some problem .

SAMADHI

Its the eighth stage of yoga, The word Samadhi means TOMP. Then you imagined how the word fit for this section, before going to this chapter one should knows about how the past deed entered in to our body ,with one mythological story .

Whenever the birth will take our poorva karma is activate in the child, the SAT VAYU is one of the responsible for our crying. the SATVAYU is deeply sleeping in our kundali mandalam, when the birth take place it first reaches the kapalam and produced crying ,any modern science doe's not described about the first crying of the child in mother womb the foetus is active ,moving ,rotate but not respirator and crying ,the ayurveda only deals about this function of the chid .

In vaishnavam thre is one acharyas called as SADAKOPAN when he birth he is not crying ,he control this SATVAYU ,so he called as SADAKOPAN ,at the time of birth taken this sad vayu is activate all our past deeds in our present life .

Well, come to our SAMADHI ANGA IS EIGHT PART OF THE YOGA after completion of the seven stages the person enters in SAMADHI part, he ready to attain the salvation, our past deed activity reduced and enter in the great cosmic power.

The cosmic power of the YOGI WILL PRODUCED some power to the human body so they called as SIDDHAR there are eighteen number of sidhar in India .they got the divine power called as ASTAMA SIDDHIS {EIGHT SUPER NATURAL POWER}.

When super natural power attained in Samadhi stage ,their body become immortal ,and this place is called as JEEVA SAMADHI ,some places in Tamilnadu very popular by this divine power.

So I got interested about the super natural people and miracle ,wonders they performed in the ancient days I deeply involved and do research activity about them ,for all miracle work there is one platform is there ,that is YOGA SCIENCE .in that yoga they attain eight supernatural power such as ,

1-ANIMA

2-MAHIMA

3-KARIMA

4-LAHIMA

5-PRATHI

6-PRAKAMIYAM

7-ESATHUVAM

8-VASITHUVAM

Is one of the supernatural power taken by ancient sages of India ,the etymology of the word anima is atom ,the person taken the position of atom like minute structure , for example the great sage AGASTHYAR is in the form of dwarf only ,but his power is balanced the tilted earth ,for request of lord Siva.

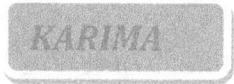

The etymology of the word MAHIMA means large structure like mountain ,in mahabarartham at the time of BAGAVAT GITHA demonstration by lord KRISHNA he take this visvaroopam structure, the great agasthyiar sage also get visvaroopam in crossing the vindhya mountain region .

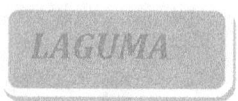

The etymology of the word karima is increasing the weight .there no change of physical position the weight of the body gets increased more than normal level.

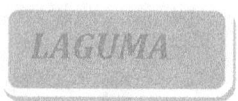

Means weight less nature, in this position the person can able to fly in sky .

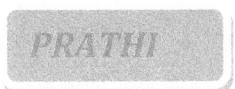

PRATHI

In this stage whatever the thoughts and wishes of the followers and devotee of the sages, he will able to fulfil their wishes and thought.

PRAKANIYAM

In this stage a person can able to transform all power to his student are follower .at the last stage of age before going to death .the senior person and his direct follower sit for long time in yoga .meditation ,after several hour of meditation the master transfer all his power to his student ,to continue his philosophy in the world.

ESATHUVAM

He is keeping all power equal to divine ,he can able to create or he can able to destroy anything .here I tell one story about GUHAI NAMACHYVAYAM,

He is one of the great sage who lived in THIRUVANNAMALAI MOUNTAIN ,one day his mutt some person are carry a dead body ,they mistakenly identified he is in un consciousness ,so they put the dead man in front of the sage he know about the situation ,and his super natural power he give life to that person, this message spread like wild fire full of city .after a week some youth are took carry his one of friends in front of SAGE ,BUT the great sage inference that they are acting to test his divine power .so he tell to them that he was already dead nobody cant help him .suddenly all friends are laughing and touch the person to awakening ,but he really died .

So creation and destruction is the divine power attained by the sages is called as EASTHUVAM.

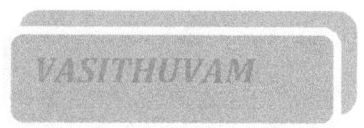

All living beings are attracted towards the person, there many evidence are ready to show this term. The sages are friendly with lion, tiger etc .

For attain above the super natural power the **YOGA FOUNDATION IS ESSENTIAL,** yoga not only for physical body as well as good mental balance has to be provided by the yoga ,

Dear reader apart from pathanjali many authors are explain in different view about **YOGA ORIGIN AND DEVELOPMENT** ,but here I, think this explanation is enough to our reader ,because the **PATHANJALLI** view is best among them ,and very simple to beginners at any age ,SO NOW WE HAVE YOU READY TO MOVE THE POSTURAL LESSONS.

ASANAM

In eight fold of yoga the **ASANAM** got a major significance roll, it nearly compared to present day **GYMNASTICS** but it entirely differs from it. in recent days it was practiced all over the world ,from toddler to old person , they have perform this postural exercise ,in school competition ,national level competition it can be conducted ,but in olden days it was very difficult. only the **INDAIN MEDICINE PHYHCIAN** and yogis ,sages ,saint are well known about this postural exercise .this was true because they only know abut the procedure and benefits and contraindication .today even the person doesn't know about the body and its constitution ,anatomy and physiology, they can do this posture .

But it is not advisable ,before entering into the postural practice one must know about **YOGA** and its origin ,development etc ,and in second stage he must under gone the **YAMA** ,and **NIYAMA** practice in his life at least try to follow the **YAMA** and **NIYAMA** which was I explain in the yoga chapter. Then only the fruits of yoga comes to our hand otherwise it can't possible.

For one example I say without proper oral cleaning and bowel cleaning one who perform this posture will lead some indigestion disorder, and some neurological disorder .some person sitting in posture and they think about their enemies ,and revenging mind will lead to some anxiety disorder.

So dear reader the proper gateway is essential for postural performance, for this reason the great , **SAGE PATHANJALI** put this posture in third number .

Sthira-sukham-asanam ||46||

स्थिर सुख मासनम् ॥४६॥

STHIRAM –STEADY

SUKHAM-COMFORTABLE

ASANAM- POSTURE

In pathanjali sutram ,the second chapter named as SADHANA PADAM the verses number 46 ,he tell about the posture in a single line .which seating pose is steady and making you comfortable and pleasure is called as POSTURE or asanam.

The etymology of the word ASANAM is come from ,the Sanskrit word, is given the meaning of- TO SIT DOWN ,in every animal origin in the world, after the routine work they will going to take rest in a shadow ,under the tree or the shadow of a building, or shed all animal origin are supported by four limps ,so they can't get tired easily .but the human is different from others ,he give separate function lower limp to walk and upper limp for other action, so he can easily get tired ,so he want to take rest compulsory ,so he sit with his buttocks part in other animal like cow ,elephant are unable to sit with buttocks ,the animal can take rest with abdominal part only. so the word sitting is very suitable for human beings .

In Indus VALLEY CIVILIZATION period has provide some valuable information about the postural has practiced in those days .the broken earthen pots symbols, and meditation symbols of lord PASUPATHY with three head, has provide the evidence of ASANAM has practiced in HARAPPA AND MAHANJADHARO period also .the time period of sindhu river valley is more than three thousand seven fifty years old.

WHY IT GET IMPORTANT

AS A SPIRITUAL SIGNIFICANTS:

The importance of the yoga is to attain the salvation purpose ,has demonstrated in the HINDHU religion .according to some tradition in Hindu religion they buried the dead man in to padmasanam posture ,Many sages are buried in this method only .

Apart from Hindu religion the posture is performed in the BUDHIST and JAINISH religion also .the LORD BUDHA is present in LOTUS POSTURE only ,he born as a son of a king ,he went out his palace to search for the wisdom .after six years meditation in the bible tree he attain wisdom .

In Jainism also the PARSWANADHAR also went for search the wisdom and get wisdom. In TAMIL one poem collection named as NATRINAI it s more than two thousand year old .they mentioned that the JAINIST SAGE are always present in the posture only .likewise the ASANAM got significant role in the devotional aspect .

PROVIDE GOOD PHYSICAL HEALTH

And there is one more important role of the ASANAM is one of the form of our daily physical exercise , To maintain our good health and avoid your risk of health problems, the doctors are recommend a minimum of 30 minutes of physical activity .is more beneficial for all , days and all age groups.

The posture will help to your burn calories that you store from eating throughout the day and—it can be done in the form of padmasanam, trikonasanam, vajrasanam etc. Providing opportunities for children to be active early on puts them on a path to good physical and mental health. It's never too late to jumpstart a healthy lifestyle.

PROVIDE GOOD MENTAL HEALTH

ASANAM not only for spiritual and physical health. it has provide lot of good effect to mental health, first it reduce the stress and strain ,improve the mental concentration and memory power ,reduced the anxiety and parkinsonism diseases ,the anxiety is reduced ,some person always irritant and anger ,short tempered also reduced by this postural exercise .

According to world health organization the good health defined as , "a state of complete physical, mental and social wellbeing and not merely the absence of disease or infirmity in simple form Health may be defined as the ability to adapt and manage physical, mental and social challenges throughout life. THE POSTURAL HAS FULLFILLED THE WHO AIM WITH OUT ANY DOUBLT.

TYPES OF ASANAM

The postural exercise can be classified in to the way of performance ,for example

SITTING TYPE –PADMASANAM

STANDING TYPE –TADA ASANAM

RECLING TYPE –SAVASASNAM

INVERTED TYPE –SIRASANAM

BALANCING TYPE-KUKUDAASANAM ,MAYURA ASANAM

HIP OPENING TYPE-GOMUKASANAM etc are some type of posture ,the modern authors and it classified in recent days ,in oldest text there is no classification found ,for reader information only I have give this types .

DO"S AND DONTS

When going to practice the posture ,some do's and don'ts is essential because this is related to body and mind ,even small mistake will lead to some harmful effect, so here I have to mention some essential steps you have to practice in your postural exercise .

Do's

1-bramaha Murtha time is preferable which has to come early morning 3-45am to before sun rise .there is one proverb follow the sun remove all the problem ,so early morning time suitable for *YOGA* practices .

2-eliminate faeces and urine is essential .

3-after bath is necessary but this postural will produce some sweating so usually before bath is conducted .

4- if you need take some warm milk with mild sugar .

5-take proper sleep in night ,without sound sleep no one can perform any work ,so good sleep is essential for all work.

6-good ventilation and proper light in needed .the sun rays place is suitable.

7-the floor must be in equal level ,free from thorns and small stones .

8-free from noise pollution ,without any disturbance is essential .

9-don't suppress natural urges during the posture performance.

10-please rhythmically perform the yoga ,not perform very fast .

11-please dry to take vegetarian meals .when take non –vegetarian food it induced RAJASIKA mind ,so, violence activity will be created.

1-women during menstrual time

2-during 2nd and 3rd trimester of pregnancy.

3-avoid smoke and alcohol and narcotics item.

4-rigorus and fast movement .

5-without good sleep .

6-after intake of meals .and water.

7-during natural calamity.

8-body illness due to pathological and accident .

9-dont take immediate bath .give rest for 30minutes after you have to bath.

10-witout proper guidance in PRANAYAMA {breathing exercise }no one should perform along with posture ,because some time it awakening the KUNDALINI POWER .it may lead to some risk .

11-recently undergone any surgery .

DRESS -CODE

Before entering into the yoga practices A person should be careful about to his dresses. Dear reader you have to watch some internet and video channel those who describe about the yoga they have to wear sexual sense stimulating Apparels, these dresses are not suitable for yoga posture and practices of yoga.

why I am telling like this , the posture is not only for goodness of the body as well as the mind also get benefited by this posture, this types of dress which has to produce some sexual stimulation to other yoga practitioner , who has practice near to you. so the selection of the dress is essential for yoga practitioner .that dress is in free in size. which has to cover all parts of the body . that dress must be clean and free from bad odor . some person using body spray and perfume it may be irritant to some others. So, you have to avoid irritant odor and perfume in group exercise and posture performance

DIETICS METHOD

1-please take vegetable foods .

2-please avoid animal origin food due to it induced **RAJASIKA GUNAM** in mind .

3- avoid fried food item and semi cooked food item.

4-some foods are induced thirst so one may avoid it .

5-excessive food intake ,should be avoid .

6-please avoid spicy .gravy masala food .

7-take warm water or warm milk mild sugar .

8-take **ALMOND** and **CASHEW NUT**.

9-take water in empty stomach when awakening from bed is good for ideal health.

10-dark green vegetables and leaf are enriched with magnesium and zinc it boost up our immunity and concentration power.

11-take butter ,and melted ghee is ideal for good health.

12-the readymade. and backed food should be avoid.

13-take vegetable soup in evening time with mild pepper it reduced excessive kapha accumulation in our body.

14-take butter milk with asafoetida powder it will reduce the flatulence and excessive gas accumulation in stomach.

15-atleast in yearly two time should undergone purgation therapy it will beneficial and prevent forthcoming diseases .

16-take banana ,water melon ,whole wheat grains are taken .

17-take sprouted grains .

18-take meals and food when hungry is started .without hungry don't take any meals.

1-SOORIYA NAMASKARA (SUN SALUTATION)

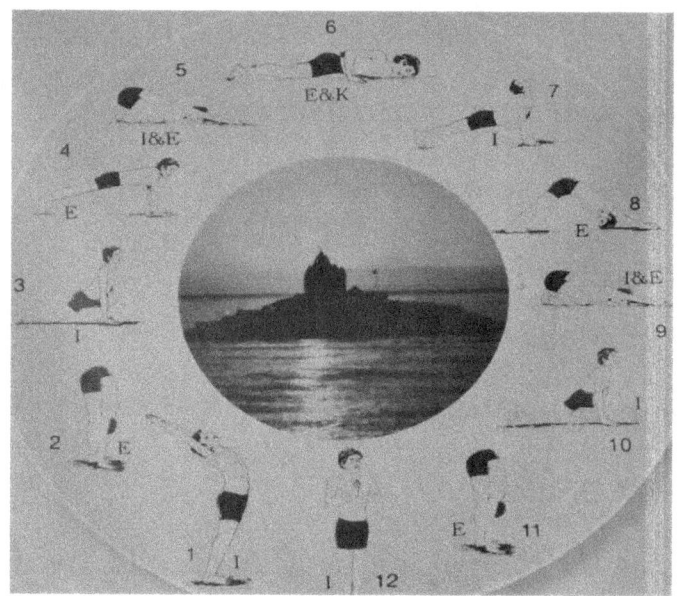

WHAT IS SOORYA NAMASKAR

The word meaning sooriya namaskar means SUN SALUTATION, in Hindu religion sun is worshiped as GOD. The sun is primary source of energies in our solar system. Various ancient scholar, sages are praised the sun ,.sooriya puranam that means the ancients literature which dealt & narrate about sun.

The sun god another name was ADHITHYAS, he travel with chariot of seven horses and single wheel .the seven horse represent seven days. his wife name is USHA and PRATHYUSHA ,his sun name lord saneeswarar .lord HANUMAN is his student .

Today modern science also described the health benefit of sun, follow the sun is one of the famous proverb in India, early morning awakening is very helpful to maintain our healthy life .In morning time sun rays are very much useful for health system. it improve our circulation also. when doing in early morning with empty stomach it give appetite ,unused calories are burned .sun salutation is one of best aerobic tools ,both body and main work together, during this sun salutation inhaling the pure air is give refreshment throughout the day.

Procedure

1-PRAYER POSTURE

This one is the first stage sun salutation, join the two lower limps together, with relaxed standing posture ,breath normally with concentrated mind. and slowly lift the arm of joining the two palm ,and the palms placed on the chest ,like prayer to god of sun.

2-RAISED ARM POSTURE

Maintain the above posture and slowly lift the arm by very close up with ears ,at this time two palms are united and straightened .after that slowly bend the arm behind the body by slightly bending the hands.

3-BENDING DOWNWARD POSTURE

After complete the second stage, slowly bend the body by exhaling the air from the mouth, and touch the ground below the foot with palm.

4-EQUESTRIAN POSTURE

After completing the third stage, slowly take the right leg behind the body to touch knee of right limp to touch the ground. The left leg will placed with folding the knee it touches the chest.

5-DANDASASNA

After completion of fourth stage .slowly the left leg back to the body ,equal to the level of right leg. and placed the palm on the ground and lift he body with help of hand and the leg remain as it is .

6-ASTANGA POSTURE

After completion of fifth posture, slowly down the hand by touch the chest on the ground.

two palm and chest are in equal position ,then slowly raise the buttocks region by knee touches the ground, the face is forward towards the earth..

Two palm ,two foot two knee chest and chin touch the ground level these eight parts touch on the earth is called as astanga posture.

7-BHUJANGASASANAM

After completion of sixth stage ,slowly down the waist region to the earth, and lift the chest region by pressing the palm on the earth and straightening the elbow ,and face the head in upright position and maintained for two to three minute time duration.

8-ADHOMUKAHA ASANAM

In this posture again you have to raise the hip region during this time your foot will forwarded step .make the body in a triangular shape .and face your toes .

9-EQUESTRIAN POSTURE

After completing the eighth stage, slowly take the right leg behind the body to touch knee of right limp to touch the ground. The left leg will placed with folding the knee it touches the chest.

10-HASTHAPADAASANAM

Stand in a erect position, slowly bend down the hip and touch earth with palm ,the face is towards facing the knee and maintain for two three minute duration.

11-HASTHAM UTTHANA ASANAM

After completion of tenth stage slowly stand in erect position, and lift the arm and bend backwards position during this posture the waist also slightly bended.

12-TADAASANAM

After completion of eleventh posture stand in erect position, and put the arms in downward direction ,and relaxed the body ,take deep breath for three to five minutes ,and come to normal after five minutes .

Repeat this cycle of asana for two to three times depend upon your ability.

Benefits of sun salutation

First one days it's difficult to do this procedure after a week its come under a routine life.

It is very useful to maintain and strengthen muscle and joint system.

Reduced un wanted calories which will helpful to reduced the body weight.

When proper inhale and exhale the expand and contraction function of lung maintained in a good way.

Early morning watching the sun is very beneficial to our eyes.

The sun salutation increase the appetite due its bending of abdomen and unwanted flatulence, deposited stools are removed from our body.

Constipation get relieves.

In early morning when does this sun salutation mild sweating is comes out and give skin soften and enhance the skin beauty.

Its one of the good remedies for females those who suffering from menstrual problem, dysmenoreah, induce the ovulation, and help to release ovum from ovary.

It will improve the physical and mental balance.

There is one proverb in Tamil language say **KAN KETTA PINNAR SOORIYA NAMASKARAM** in proverb say the importance sun salutation for eyes .like this every one should do this sun salutation it will provide good health for us .

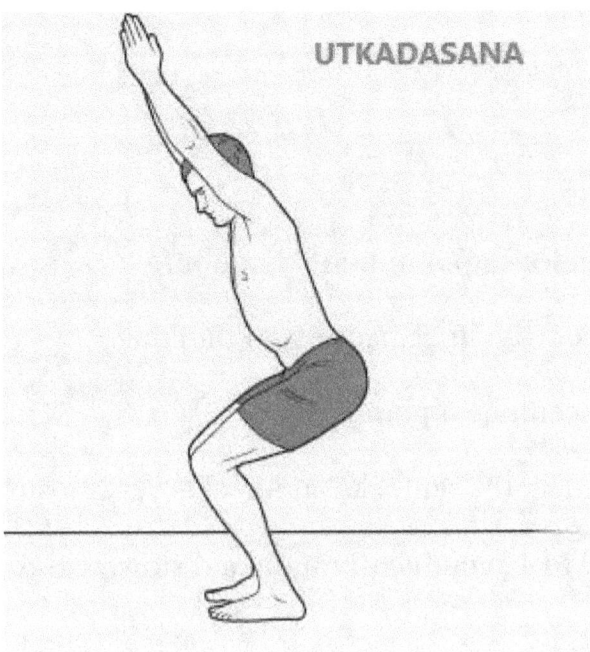

UTKADASANA

DEFINATION

The word meaning of UTKADASANA is joining of two Sanskrit word, one is utkata the other one is asana, these two words joining and provide the name UTKATASANA, UTKATA gives meaning is furious, or intense or powerful, and asana meaning is posture or seat.

Some latest scholar says that, they correlate with modern chair position, in my view sitting on chair position not provide the name *UTKADA OR FURIOUS, in* word meaning also it is not easy to do ,it is very hard furious one to do.

The exact posture of utkatasana are illustrated as painting in Mysore palace by krishnaraja wodeyar.a man folding his knee bend and sit his heel to touch the bottom of the back region. it is very hard to sit ,regular practise only achieve this asanam otherwise unable to possible to do it .

procedure

1-stand and erect position.

2-take breath and exhale it for 2 to 3 minute duration.

3-calm your mind and free from imagination and thinking,

Focus your mind and concentrate a point.

Slowly sit by folding the knee, the buttocks and heel is very closure and in a straight line.

Remaining sit calm for 10 to 15 minute duration and slowly relax the leg and try to stand slowly.

Don't stand quickly.

Stand erectly and relax by breathing and slowly move

This posture is difficulty in first few days, after some days proper training it should be very easy to practice ,

Some scholars are doing other method it is very easy one but there is no authentically evidence for this type of sitting posture.

Stand erectly by calm mind as described in previous method.

Joined the both heels.

And lift the arm forward jointly.

Slowly try to sit in chair position without the presentation of chair.

First it is very difficult to practice and sit.

After proper training this only very easy and less difficult to compare previous one.

Benefit

Provide strength to spine and waist region.

Pelvic muscle get strengthen.

Calve muscle hip muscle thigh muscles are get nourished and well developed.

Air holding capacity of lung got increased.

Relive from abdominal gas and flatulence.

Body balance function got improved.

Stimulate the live r by increasing the abdominal pressure it give good appetite also.

Contra indication

Those who affected by severe arthritis.

High Blood pressure.

Cardiac problem.

3- TRIKONASANA

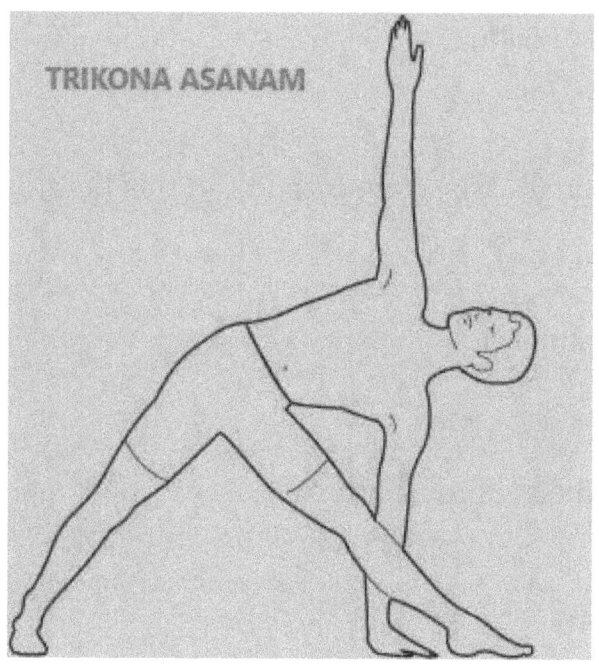

TRIKONA ASANAM

DEFINATION

   The word   trikonasana contain a combination of three word provide trikonasana .the one is tri means three ,Kona means angle and last one asana means posture. So the three words jointly formed and make the word trikonasana .its one of the important asana, make our body in to three angular postures is called as trikonasana. There various sub type of asana are thre in this main asana, the reader kindly avoid them in initial stage and do this main posture only.

Procedure

The suitable time for this posture morning and evening ,is ideal .mainly the person with empty stomach ,and evacuate stools and urine .particularly free bowel movement is mainly presented when doing this posture .

The person who planned do perform this asana ,select one calm place with proper air and sun light .particularly the ideal time of the sunrise. he spread bed sheet or yoga sheet available in the market .stand on the yoga sheet with calm mind ,and take breathe and exhale for three minutes ,and stand up straight ,slightly wide up the leg ,without bending the knee ,completely turn the right foot outside the body and the left foot less than 45 degrees inside the body, the arms are spread out to sides ,and slowly bend sideward's towards right side of the body and touch the foot with palm of the right hand ,meanwhile the time left hand will straight up wards for this posture you should keep up this, second to one minute duration ,like that left side should be done for the same time duration.

Repeat this process for ten to fifteen minute duration.

Benefit of this posture

1-the hips and pelvic muscle are get strengthened and its prevent the fat deposition in the abdomen.

2-pelvic organ like uterus bladder are supplied by good blood supply and nourished well.

3-inter rips muscle get strengthen and lung capacity get increased, UN used surface of lungs are fulfilled by pure air.

4-human is only mammals to keep stand position by two legs other mammals are supported by four limps ,so the weight should be all focused in hip region only ,the lumbar vertebra which one support the hip region are get affected ,this posture will helpful for the hip and lumbar region.

5-it stimulate the abdominal region increase the appetite

6-in old age less physical movement, stools are getting staged in descending colon and some time in sigmoid colon it will evacuate the staged stools and free from it.

7alllimbs are worked simultaneously and it will one of the warm-up exercise.

8-it will very helpful to reduce the body weight.

PRECAUTION

1-those who are pregnant.

2-those affected by cardiac problem.

3-any undergone surgery.

4-long duration bedridden.

5-after taking heavy meals and empty stomach.

4- BHUJANGAASANAS

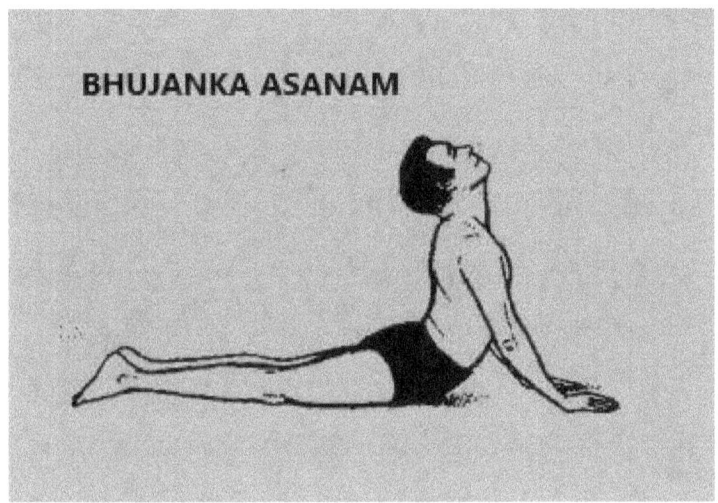

BHUJANKA ASANAM

DEFINATION

Dear readers today am going to illustrate about BHUJANGA ASANA ,it joining of two word one is bhujanga and other one is asanam ,the *bhujanga word means copra* with expand of its hood asana means posture .the asana resemble like copra pose .one of the ancient text *HATHA YOGA PRADHIPIKA* illustrate this asana and *SRITTATVANIDHI* also mentioned this type of asana and called as *SERPAASANAM or serpantpose in English.*

PROCEDURE

When going to perform this asana early morning is suitable time ,after elimination of stool and urine ,take right place to perform this posture, without any disturbance ,.spread the bed sheet and yoga mate ,and stand with a focused mind with concentration ,take deep breath and exhale do this for at least three to five minutes.

Lying down when the belly towards earth.

After that slowly lifting the head with the support of hands it usually on the side of the trunk.

Meanwhile time you should inhale the air slowly.

When raisin the body the elbow not bend, straightening the hand and lift the body in upward direction

While raising the body the legs are straightening with slowly bend the knees in this time you should exhale the air slowly.

When down the body you try inhale slowly and in upward position exhale the air slowly.

Repeat the process for ten to fifteen minute In upward direction try to maintain at least 45 second to one minute during the session you should hold the air .

Benefit of this posture

1-among the posture it one for the rejuvenating posture .

2-it crease the lung capacity.

3-holdind the air in the lungs is benefit for asthmatic patient .

4-when children practise this posture it is very beneficial to them it will increase appetite and achievement of good height.

5-the shoulder and arm get beneficial increased the strength of arms and hip region.

6-it reduces the abdominal fat.

7-expand the chest level due to holding of air.

8-when inhale the air in morning time it keep us free from stress and fatigue, it will rejuvenate our body.

9-improve the blood circulation all over the body.

10-tones the abdominal walls and prevent the herniation disorder.

11-make the spine bone strengthens.

Precaution

1-those who are pregnant.

2-recently got fractured in chest and rips.

3-recently undergone any abdominal surgery.

4-those affected by hernia   disorder.

5-abnormal high blood pressure and cardiac problem people should be avoided.

5-SARVANGA ASANAM

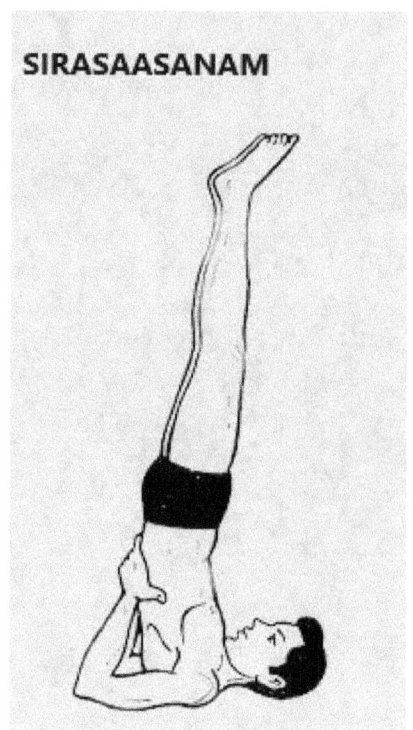

SIRASAASANAM

DEFINATION

Dear readers today am going to illustrate about sarvanga asana .the word sarvanga contain two words jointly one is sarvam and other one is angam ,sarvam means entire and anga means limps ,asanam means posture these three word jointly formed sarvangaasanam that means entire all limps or total body involved in this asanam .so it is called as sarvangaasanam. According to hatha yoga its none of the important yoga, the entire body get beneficed by this posture

PROCEDURE

It is not like ordinary posture, one who wants to do this posture .mainly the person with empty stomach ,and evacuate stools and urine .particularly free bowel movement is mainly presented when doing this posture .Small amount of water may be drink, ,take right place to perform this posture, without any disturbance ,.spread the bed sheet and yoga mate ,and stand with a focused mind with concentration ,take deep breath and exhale do this for at least three to five minutes.

Then slowly lie down on the mate like savaasanas, and relaxed the body, slowly inhale the breath.

Then placed the palm downward position facing to the earth, then slowly lift the both leg in upward direction 90degree from the hip level.

Then slowly exhale and inhale the breath and Waite for thirty second duration.

Then again exhale the air then slowly raised the body from the trunk level meanwhile the leg is slightly bended towards head.

Then again straighten the whole body place the head and neck on the earth the hand will support the hip region, exactly in 90 degree position maintain this posture up to five to seven minute duration, the reader should note one experienced candidate will do this asana for more than ten minute and not exceeding fifteen minute duration.

During this posture the eye sight should be focused to the toe will improve the eye sight .then slowly relaxed and down the limp slowly ,and relaxed then take rest for ten minute then come to normal position.

Benefit of this posture

When do this posture the blood supply get increased the hip region, the varicose vein disorder get reduced and prevent the same disorder.

Body weight get balanced by this asana .some of us have different body weight our body divided in to two parts from hip to leg and other one is hip two head ,these type of weight disorder get balanced by this posture.

The human only mammals to using two limps so the gravitational force all pelvic organs are placed in the pelvic region and lack of space for the internal organ so this function of this organ get affected .when do this posture all organs get relaxed and do their function well. And normal gravitational pressure gets maintained.

Uterine prolapsed to get it right, and strengthen the uterine ligaments and uterine muscles,

Prevent and cure the haemorrhoids' disorder.

Some authors give opinion that this posture will cure or prevent thyroidal disorder.

It nourishes the inner organ and rejuvenates the body.

PRECAUTION

1-Those who are suffered by head and neck disorder.

2-During menstrual time.

3-Suffering from liver cirrhosis or hepato megaly or spleeno megaly disorder .

4-those who are pregnant.

5-those affected by cardiac problem.

6-any undergone surgery.

7-long duration bedridden.

8-after taking heavy meals and empty stomach.

9-cervical bone disorder.

6- VRIKSHAASANAM

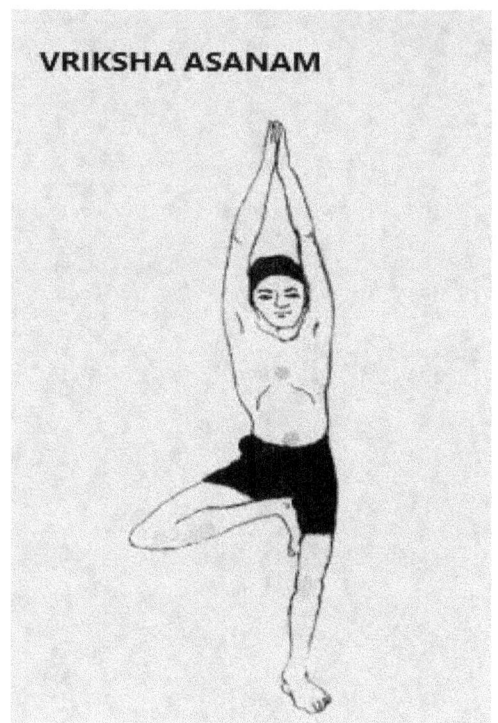

VRIKSHA ASANAM

DEFINATION

Dear reader today I am going to described about **VRIKSHAASANA** it is the joining of two word one is ***VRIKSHA or vriksham it denote to tree*** and asana means posture .a seventeenth century text ***GHERANDA SAMHITHA*** had described this posture, and the famous stone carving in **mahabalipuram** which belongs to seventh century had described this posture ,.in ancient time sages are performed this posture to attained salvation. Unlike other posture this posture is different, when doing this asana our eyes are should open to balance our weight.

When plan to do this posture select one peaceful place, devoid of noise and pollution free place. Stand on the mate or bed sheet and slowly take breath for three to five minute duration with concentration of mind,

Stand in comfortable position, slowly lift the right leg and the sole place it on the left leg which is placed on the ground.

When sole of right leg placed at any comfortable place of the left leg inner side.

Slowly move the right leg near as possible to the groin region, and placed it and equal pressure should be emitted by both limps.

The right knee should be the level of 45 degree angle level.

Relax the shoulder region and lift the both hand and palm of the hand should be joined, if it possible please perform ankuli mudra posture.

Like that should do opposite leg.

Minimum time duration for each limp should be maintained d three to five minutes duration.

BENEFIT OF THIS POSTURE

1-BODY BALANCE FUNCTION IMPROVED BY THIS POSTURE .

2-the spine and legs are get strengthened by this posture.

3-the angle joint and knee joint get much more beneficial.

4-when perform this posture we consume more oxygen, so the apex surface of lungs are filled by air .the apex surface is the main place for tuberculosis bacteria. They mainly cultivate and spread from this area only.

5-our concentration will be improved .in olden day our sages are performed this posture for obtain boon from the god.

6-it will tone the muscle of back region and chest region also.

7-the sciatica the disorder affect the degeneration of sciatic nerve due any compression or pathological reason along with any treatment do this posture it will support your health.

8-the premenstrual symptoms are reduced.

9-when doing this posture in a concentrated mind, it free from anxiety, stress, also.

10-learning function of children get improved.

CONTRAINDICATION

1-Is there any recent fracture in lower limp.

2-recently undergone any surgery.

3-afeected by any central nervous system disorder .

4-per who suffered from arthritis and balancing disorder like vertigo or giddiness are advised to no do this posture.

5-surrounding area is free from hazardous material it may cause injury to us.

7- <u>TADASANAM</u>

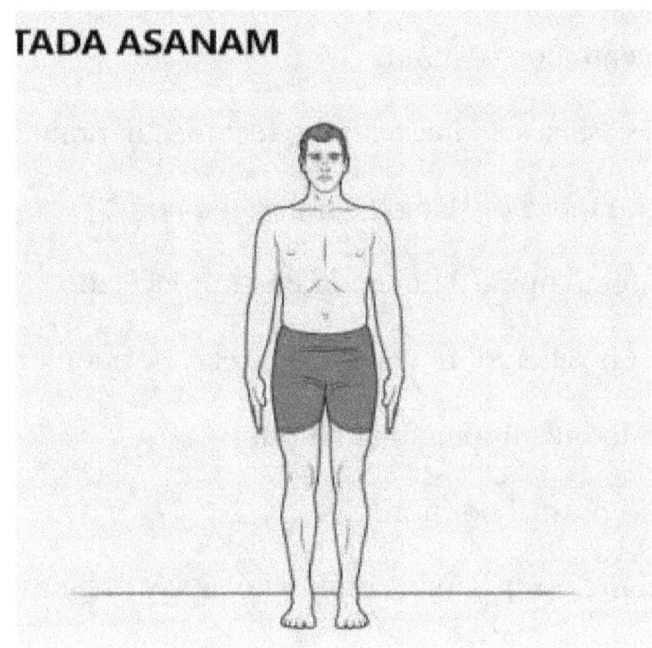

TADA ASANAM

Dear readers today am going to illustrate about TADAASANAM in etymology the word
TADA means the MOUNTAIN asana means posture so it called as mountain posture or
tadaasanam, in some literature this posture is mentioned as samasthithi asana ,word meaning
for sama means stable or maintain the equilibrium ,sthithi means standings and asana means
posture so the word meaning is maintain the equilibrium in standing position ,it is one of the
simple asana even children's or beginners will perform his posture ,it is very easy perform .

HATHA YOGA one of the ancient texts mentioned about this asana.

PROCEDURE

When plan to do this posture select one peaceful place, devoid of noise and pollution free place. Stand on the mate or bed sheet and slowly take breath for three to five minute duration with concentration of mind,

When perform this asana standing with the feet together on the mate,.

Down the hand And move the hand lateral to the body,

And face the palm in to upward direction like our face appeared.

And maintain erect position of the body with relax position of mind.

Maintain up to ten to fifteen minute duration.

And slowly come to normal position.

Various opinion about this posture, some scholar say to lift the hand in upward direction,

and some say interlock the fingers and keep upwards above the head level .but my opinion is the simple one procedure above mentioned by me is simple and authentically .

BENEFIT OF THIS POSTURE.

1-it is proven one to reduce our abdominal fat.

2-this posture burned out all under arms fat.

3-get relief from stress and anxiety.

4-it improves the body posture.

5-when regular postures this makes our knees, angles, get strengthen.

6-heigt will increased

7-our digestive and nervous system are regulated.

CONTRA INDICATION

1-Affected by previous nervous disorder .

2-Loss of sleep.

3-Head ache.

4-Is there any recent fracture in lower limp.

5-Those who are suffered by head and neck disorder .

6-During menstrual time.

8- NAVAASANAM

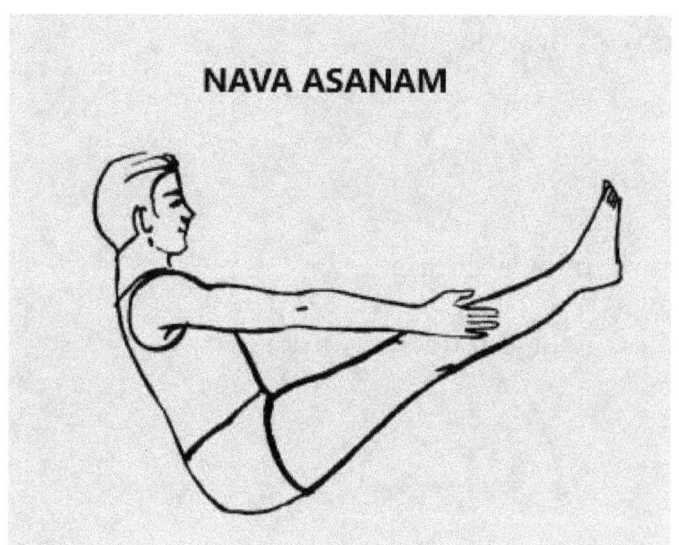

NAVA ASANAM

DEFINATION

The word NAVASANAM is also called by another name *NAUKA ASANAM* the word meaning of NAUKA is boat asana means posture, the posture which will looks like boat is called as nauka asana it is divided in to two sub types NAUKA ASANAM and other one is **PARIPURANANAVASANAM** that means complete or full boat posture .in SANSKRIT language the word NAVA or NAUKA is given meaning of boat.

PROCEDURE

Like sarvanga asana , It is very difficult one, not a ordinary posture, one who wants to do this posture .mainly the person with empty stomach ,and evacuate stools and urine .particularly free bowel movement is mainly presented when doing this posture .Small amount of water may be drink, ,take right place to perform this posture, without any disturbance ,.spread the bed sheet and yoga mate ,and stand with a focused mind with concentration ,take deep breath and exhale do this for at least three to five minutes.

Then slowly lie down on the mat, like savaasanas, and relaxed the body, slowly inhale the breath.

The whole body bend in to V shape slowly.

The buttocks are placed on the earth.

The two arms hold the middle part of the thigh and keep it for ten to fifteen minute duration.

Slowly come to normal stage.

Previous mentioned pre caution should be noted.

BENEFITS

1-Internal organ are got strength.

2-Abdominal muscle are got strengthen.

3-Blood supply is profusely supply to pelvic region, and internal pelvic organ are got nourished.

4-Any person affected by sciatica inter vertebral disc problem in sacrum lumbar joint they get beneficial by this posture,

5-it relieve the constipation and flatulence, the staged stools are eliminated,.

6-in the gall bladder bile's are stored in long time they may be crystallised, again deposition of bile liquid on the crystallisation particle it will become in to stone ,it take long time to become the gall stone ,when pressure given in gall bladder the stored bile liquid are eliminated . And prevent gall bladder stone.

CONTRAINDICATION

1-Those who are suffered by hip and leg disorder or fracture.

2-During menstrual time.

3-Suffering from liver cirrhosis or hepato megaly or spleenomegally disorder .

4-those who are pregnant.

5-those affected by cardiac problem.

6-any undergone abdominal surgery.

7- Bedridden.

8-after taking heavy meals and empty stomach.

9-cervical bone disorder .

9- BADHA KONA ASANAM

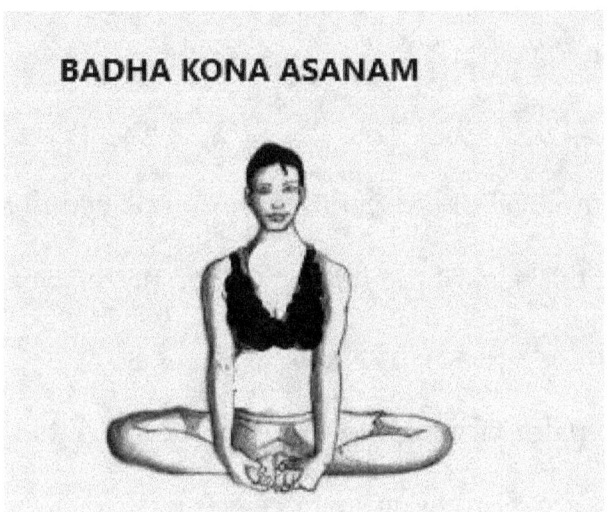

BADHA KONA ASANAM

DEFINATION:

Dear reader today i am going to described about BADHA KONA ASANA it is the joining of two word one is BADHA and other one KONA ,the word meaning for badha is bound and Kona means angle and asana means posture .so it bound angle posture or otherwise it called as copra posture .

One of the ancient texts *HATHA YOGA PRADIPIKA* in 15th centaury period had described about this posture.

it is called as copra posture due to the charmer is difficultly seated in this posture in front of the snack so it is called copra pose .

When going to perform this asana early morning is suitable time ,after elimination of stool and urine ,take right place to perform this posture, without any disturbance ,.spread the bed sheet and yoga mate ,and stand with .

Slowly sit on the mat .

First you fold the left limp, the heal of the right leg should placed near the perineum area.

Then slowly fold the left leg the heel of the left leg will be placed near to perineum.

It is very difficult to the beginners please try to sit.

Then fold the hand and the palm of the hand will be joined together.

And placed hand on the chest region, like prayer position.

BENEFIT OF THIS POSTUR

It is very benefit for internal organ like urinary bladder, uterus, and ovary.etc

It relieved the constipation, and flatulence.

This posture is one of the thigh muscles relaxing posture.

This asana is best for pregnant women, helping them normal delivery.

This asana stimulate the functioning of the reproductive system in women. Like uterus .ovary, and   tightening the uterine ligaments and prevent the uterine prolapsed It helps cure menstrual problems.

Lower part of the body got improved blood circulation.

This posture will strengthen your spine.

CONTRAINDICATION

1-Those who are suffered by hip and leg disorder or fracture.

2-During menstrual time.

<u>3</u> -those who are pregnant.

4-those affected by cardiac problem.

5-any undergone abdominal surgery.

6- Bedridden.

7-after taking heavy meals and empty stomach.

10- DHANUR ASANAM

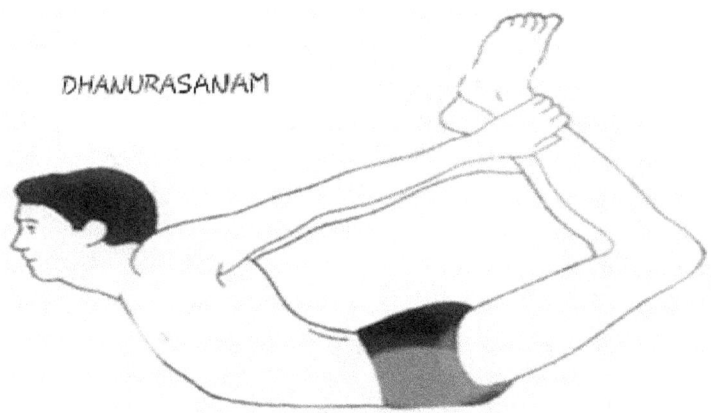

DHANURASANAM

DEFINATION

Dear reader ,welcome today i am going to illustrate about DHANURASANAM ,today in modern life and luxury life many people suffered by diabetic disorder even though young people are suffered by diabetic disorder .this posture prevent from diabetic disorder even those who suffered from diabetic this posture support them to secrete the insulin.

The word DHANURASANAM is joining of two word one is DHANUR it give meaning of bow and asana means posture so, the posture resemble like bow symbol is called as DHANUR ASANAM.

Like sarvanga asana , It is very difficult one, not a ordinary posture, one who wants to do this posture .mainly the person with empty stomach ,and evacuate stools and urine .particularly free bowel movement is mainly presented when doing this posture .Small amount of water may be drink, ,take right place to perform this posture, without any disturbance ,.spread the bed sheet and yoga mate ,and stand with a focused mind with concentration ,take deep breath and exhale do this for at least three to five minutes.

Then slowly lie down on the mat, like savaasanas, and relaxed the body, slowly inhale the breath.

Next step is slowly turn and face towards earth.

Simply in prone position.

Then slowly bend the knee and hold the ankle by hand.

Slowly bend the hip in upward movement during this session you have to lift your chest.

And face straight, upright position.

Hold the ankle with hand with strongly meanwhile time you have to exhale your breath, not inhale and hold the air.

Then slowly come to normal position keep rest three to five minute, then slowly come to supine position, then stand.

BENEFIT OF THIS POSTUR

It give compression to abdominal wall, and this pressure is reflect on pancreases, then it secrete insulin and reduce the diabetic disorder.

Some time there is obstruction in common bile duct it lead to diabetic disorder, this will also cured by this posture.

It will reduce the weight and prevent fat deposition in the lower abdomen,

It improve the function of the internal organ like liver, pancreas, kidney, bladder .etc

The spinal region also get strengthen by this asana.

It relieve the constipation and staged faeces and flatulence,

This posture helps to stimulate the internal reproductive organs, like uterus, ovary etc.

Regular practicing this posture wills helps to wide, chest, and shoulders.

The legs and arm muscles are got strengthened.

Menstrual discomfort also relieved by this posture regularly.

This posture will helpful to people who affect by renal disorder.

CONTRAINDICATION

People those who are suffered by cardiac problem and hypertension should not do this posture.

1-Those who are suffered by hip and leg disorder or fracture.

2-During menstrual time.

3-Suffering from liver cirrhosis or stomach ulceration are not advised do this posture.

4-those who are pregnant.

5-any undergone abdominal surgery.

6- Bedridden.

7-after taking heavy meals and empty stomach.

8-before sleep this posture usually not advised .

9-person with any renal disorder or affected by any renal calculi not advised to do this posture.

11-PADMASANAM

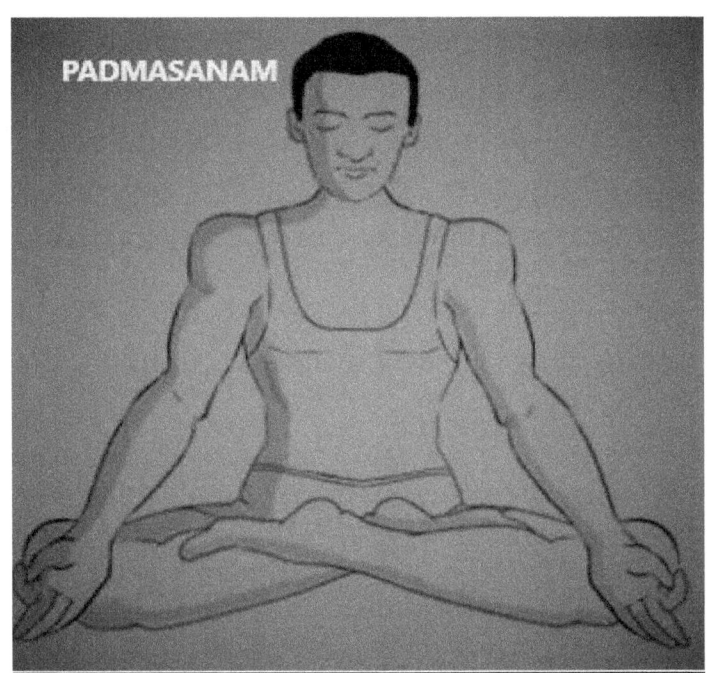

The reader those who knows about HINDHU religion they must familiar with this posture because the most worship posture of god is seat on the lotus ,the great sages they perform majestic with this posture seated on a divine lotus.

Latter in Buddhism and Jainism also the worship god seated on the lotus flower in this lotus posture,

The word meaning PADMASANAM means joining of two words one is padma is lotus and asasanam means posture so it is called as lotus posture.

Dear reader , one who wants to do this posture .mainly the person with empty stomach ,and evacuate stools and urine .particularly free bowel movement is mainly presented when doing this posture .Small amount of water may be drink, ,take right place to perform this posture, without any disturbance ,.spread the bed sheet and yoga mate ,and stand with a focused mind with concentration ,take deep breath and exhale do this for at least three to five minutes.

And slowly sit on the mat with legs stretched out in front of you while keeping the spine erect position

Slowly right knee bended and place it on the left thigh. The sole of the feet point upward and the heel is close to the groin region. Then, repeat the same step with the other leg.

With both the legs crossed and feet placed on opposite thighs, place your both palm on your sole of the feet.

BENEFITS

It is very famous posture among the HINDHU sages and great saint many god forms are in this posture only,

It will calm the mind.

Free from stress and strain.

Improve the appetite.

Sub conscious mind is awakening concentration and memory power,

Restore our energy level.

It relieved the constipation and flatulence.

CONTRA INDICATION

1-Those who are suffered by hip and leg disorder or fracture.

2-During menstrual time.

3 -those who are pregnant.

4-those affected by cardiac problem.

5-any undergone abdominal surgery.

6- Bedridden.

7-after taking heavy meals and empty stomach.

12-PASCHIMOUTTANA ASANAM

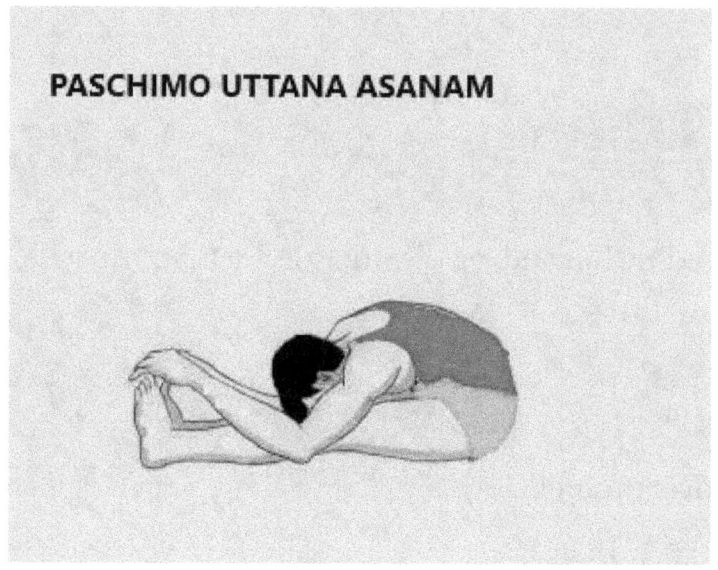

PASCHIMO UTTANA ASANAM

DEFINITION

Dear reader today am going to illustrate about paschimouttana asanam, it is a combination of three word one is **PASCHIMO** this meaning is indicate the west direction. in normally a person should stand to facing the son ,it is eastern direction ,his opposite direction is west that means his back region .and the word.

UTTANA means superficial seated its opposite is *GAMPIRAM is deep seated one* ,so the word meaning of PASCHIMOUTTANA is the back region is superficial to find ,that means the person deep stretched bending forward position, and ASANAM means posture ,so it called as deep stretched bending forwarded position is called as *PASCHIMOUTTANA ASANAM.*

It is very difficult one, not a ordinary posture, one who wants to do this posture .mainly the person with empty stomach ,and evacuate stools and urine .particularly free bowel movement is mainly presented when doing this posture .Small amount of water may be drink, ,take right place to perform this posture, without any disturbance ,.spread the bed sheet and yoga mate ,and stand with a focused mind with concentration ,take deep breath and exhale do this for at least three to five minutes.

Sit on the mat in a comfortable position.

and stretch your legs comfort ability .

Then you have to stretch your hand parallel to the leg.

Then you have to bend forwarded slowly without produce any spasm in the muscle .

Then you have try to catch your two toes with by palm, the elbow is placed side of the knee and note it the elbow is slightly bended.

Keep it for two to three minute duration, meanwhile time you should do wave breathe only not deep breath take place here.

Then slowly get in to normal position, and come to standing position.

BENEFITS

This asana is mainly helpful for those who affected by diabetic mellitus disorder because the entire abdomen get mild pressure and it induce to secrete the insulin from pancreas .

And other internal abdominal organ got benefited.

Reduce the belly fat,

Some people got breathing, they unable to perform any work .like this people this posture is very beneficial,

It will increase the appetite and burn excessive cholesterol which deposited in the body.

The ovaries are stimulated and reduced the infertility and menstrual problem.

It improves the respiratory functions.

CONTRA INDICATION

This posture is produce d some pressure to the abdominal cavity and some strain work needed to perform this posture ,so some pre caution is take essential ,.

People those who are suffered by cardiac problem and hypertension should not do this posture.

1-Those who are suffered by hip and leg disorder or fracture.

2-During menstrual time.

3-Suffering from liver cirrhosis or stomach ulceration are not advised do this posture.

4-those who are pregnant.

5-any undergone abdominal surgery.

6- Bedridden.

7-after taking heavy meals and empty stomach.

8-before sleep this posture usually not advised .

9-person with any renal disorder or affected by any renal calculi not advised to do this posture.

13-BAKA ASANAM

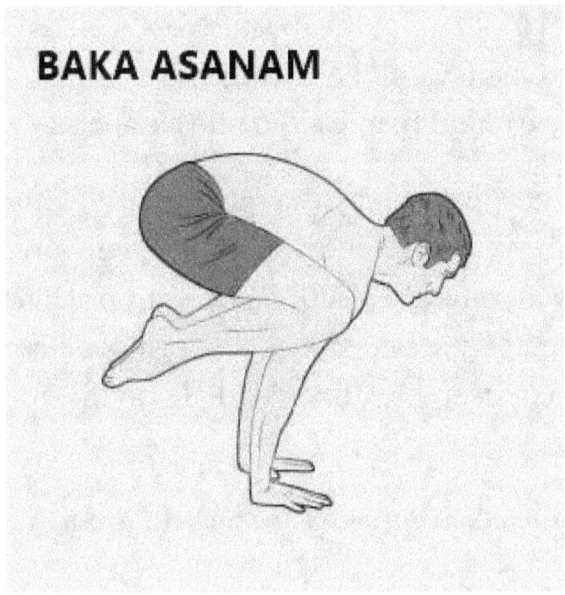

BAKA ASANAM

DEFINATION

Dear reader today am going to described about BAKA ASANAM or kaka asanam ,one of the ancient text **SRITATTVANIDHI** has described about this posture ,And *hattha ratnavali* a 17 century text has described about this posture has illustrated by lord **SIVA.**

The baka asanam is otherwise called as kaka asanam is a self balancing posture by the hand .the word meaning BAKA is crane or the word meaning kaka is crow and asanam means posture .so the posture resemble like crane or crow posture is called as baka asana or kaka asanam.

Some authors mentioned two variant of this posture one ordinary and other one is head upright position .but this asasnam is self balancing and lifting the body by two hands so its difficulty take necessary pre caution before doing this asanam.

those who wants to do this posture .mainly the person with empty stomach ,and evacuate stools and urine .particularly free bowel movement is mainly presented when doing this posture .Small amount of water may be drink, ,take right place to perform this posture, without any disturbance ,.spread the bed sheet and yoga mate ,and stand with a focused mind with concentration ,take deep breath and exhale do this for at least three to five minutes.

Then you have to place your palm on the earth, near to the feet ,

Then slowly lift the both leg simultaneously by bending the knee .

The knee is on level of the elbow and move to reach the axial region slowly.

Then face t to down the earth is one kind of asanam.

The other one lift the head and face in a upright position .

And keep it for at least two to three duration.

It is one of difficult posture during this session one try to avoid speech laugh etc,

Without proper concentration and attention advised not to perform this posture.

BENEFITS

It improve the concentration power of the mind like crane is waiting of fish in running water,

Stress and strain are remover d.

It give strengthen to arm muscle and balancing function of the body got improved.

And it is very benefited and supported for neck muscle.

CONTRAINDICATION

People those who are suffered by cardiac problem and hypertension should not do this posture.

1-Those who are suffered by hip and leg disorder or fracture.

2-During menstrual time.

3-Suffering from liver cirrhosis or stomach ulceration are not advice do this posture.

4-those who are pregnant.

5-any undergone abdominal surgery.

6- Bedridden.

7-after taking heavy meals and empty stomach.

8-before sleep this posture usually not advised .

9-person with any renal disorder or affected by any renal calculi not advised to do this posture.

14- KUKUTASANAM

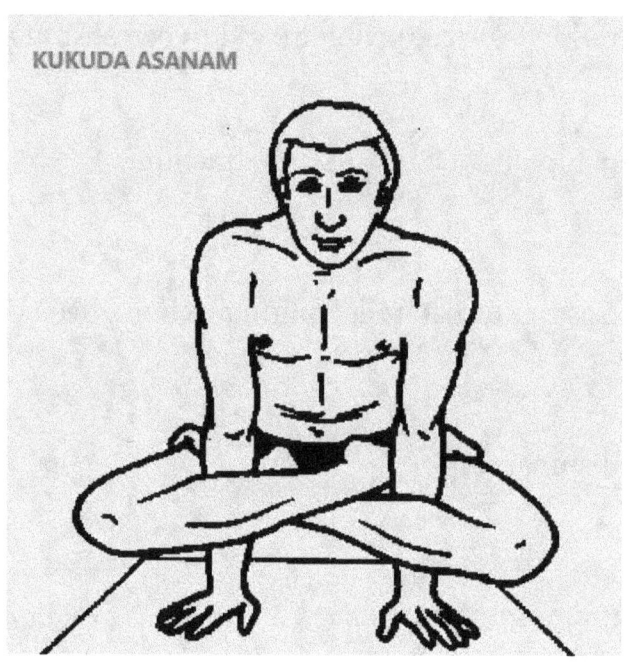

KUKUDA ASANAM

DEFINATION

The word meaning of **KUKKUTA is rooster** in English and the word ASANA means posture .the posture resemble like rooster is called as **KUKKUTASANAM**,it is one of the very classical one ,various authors are described different sub types of this asanam, but it is very difficult to perform this one ,so my advice to reader ,please follow this simple type only in the level of begins, after practising you have to done various sub posture of this type.

As like padmasanam you have to prepare initial step like wise

one who wants to do this posture .mainly the person with empty stomach ,and evacuate stools and urine .particularly free bowel movement is mainly presented when doing this posture .Small amount of water may be drink, ,take right place to perform this posture, without any disturbance ,.spread the bed sheet and yoga mate ,and stand with a focused mind with concentration ,take deep breath and exhale do this for at least three to five minutes.

And slowly sit on the mat with legs stretched out in front of you while keeping the spine erect position.

Slowly right knee bended and place it on the left thigh. The sole of the feet point upward and the heel is close to the groin region. Then, repeat the same step with the other leg.

With both the legs crossed and feet placed on opposite thighs.

Now entered one hand first in to the area of groin region and touch the earth.

Then the second hand you have to insert like that.

Now you have to lift the body by placing the palm on the earth, then you have face upwards and deep breathing ,and slowly released the air ,

Keep this position up to two to three minute's duration,

Then slowly down the body and sit in normal padmasanam, and release the hand and place it sideward's to the body by touching the knee.

This posture is very proven posture it provide strength to external genital organs .the psoas major and psoas minor muscle are get strengthened by this posture .

It relieved the constipation and flatulence,

Sciatica and degeneration of the lumbar and sacral nerve are get cured by this posture,

The for arms and arms are get strengthened by this posture.

Reduce the belly fat and tighten the abdominal wall and prevent the herniation disorder.

This posture has provide good appetite.

Uterine problem will also get subsided by this posture.

CONTRAINDICATION

People those who are suffered by cardiac problem and hypertension should not do this posture.

1-Those who are suffered by hip and leg disorder or fracture.

2-During menstrual time.

3-Suffering from liver cirrhosis or stomach ulceration are not advised do this posture.

4-those who are pregnant.5-any undergone abdominal surgery.

6- Bedridden.

7-after taking heavy meals and empty stomach.

8-before sleep this posture usually not advised .

9-person with any fracture in hand s and dislocation of the shoulder joint not advised to do this posture.

10-without proper sleep and diet you should not perform this posture .

11-befoer going to bed not advised to do this posture.

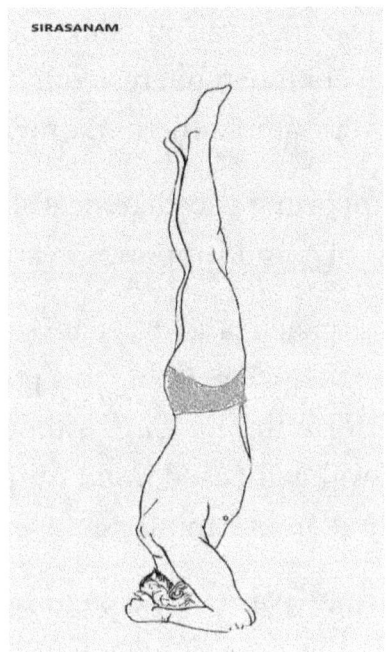

SIRASANAM

DEFINATION

In the yoga shastra the sirasasanam, got an very important roll ,it get nick name as KING OF ALL ASANAS, various samhitha 's are mentioned this posture in various name for example .in *HATHA YOGA PRADHEEPIKA* it is described as MUDRA ,In eighteenth century the text book called as *JOGA PRADEEPIKA* it was mentioned as KAPAALI ASANAS .In HATHA YOGA one of the ancient book by *HEMACHANDRA* this posture called as *DURIYOTHA ASANA or KAPALI KARANA*.

The word meaning of SIRASHASANAM is joining of two words one is SIRASH it provide the meaning of head or it is the head of all asana ,and asanam means posture so .my opinion is the word sirasasanam is practising in olden days by various name but this name is got in recent days only.

Dear reader various authors provided various sub types but it is some difficulty in earlier stage ,the young children's are very much interested in this posture but adult are feel some difficulty, so here I will explain very simple method only anyone can easily follow this one.

First of you have to choose a supporting pace like near to the wall ,because first few days we stand an inverted position need of a wall support, so carefully select a place.

mainly the person with empty stomach ,and evacuate stools and urine .particularly free bowel movement is mainly presented when doing this posture .Small amount of water may be drink, ,take right place to perform this posture, without any disturbance ,.spread the bed sheet and yoga mate ,and stand with a focused mind with concentration ,take deep breath and exhale do this for at least three to five minutes.

Then you have to touch the earth by palm of the hand by bending the body forwarded ,then slowly place the head on earth in this time simultaneously your arm will support the neck .

Now slowly up lift the whole body by given the pressure by leg then straighten the leg with the support of wall ,meanwhile time you r hand will very close to the neck the forearm will be behind the head .

Keep it for one to two minute duration.

Then slowly down the leg to earth ,and placed the knee on the earth then slowly you have to try to stand in a normal position.

BENEFIT OF THIS POSTURE

The head is the main organ it control the whole body it got a chief function and vital roll .this posture increase the blood flow to the brain and the neuron are get refresh by this posture.

It improves the hair growth.

The vision power of eye got improved.

The memory and concentrative power got improved by this posture.

Neck muscle got strengthened by this posture.

Due to anti gravity force activated in the internal organ some sediments like urea and bile are removed by this posture, so we strongly say this posture prevent the kidney stone and bile stone.

CONTRAINDICATION

Anyone have head and neck disorder they should advise not do this posture.

The person have cervical spondilities should avoid this posture.

The person has **HYPER TENSION** they should avoid this posture.

People those who are suffered by cardiac problem and hypertension should not do this posture.

1-Those who are suffered by hip and leg disorder or fracture.

2-During menstrual time.

3-Suffering from liver cirrhosis or stomach ulceration are not advised do this posture.

4-those who are pregnant.

5-any undergone abdominal surgery.

6- Bedridden.

7-after taking heavy meals and empty stomach.

8-before sleep this posture usually not advised .

9-person with any fracture in hand s and dislocation of the shoulder joint not advised to do this posture.

10-without proper sleep and diet you should not perform this posture.

11-befoer going to bed not advised to do this posture.

16-GOMUKHA ASANAM

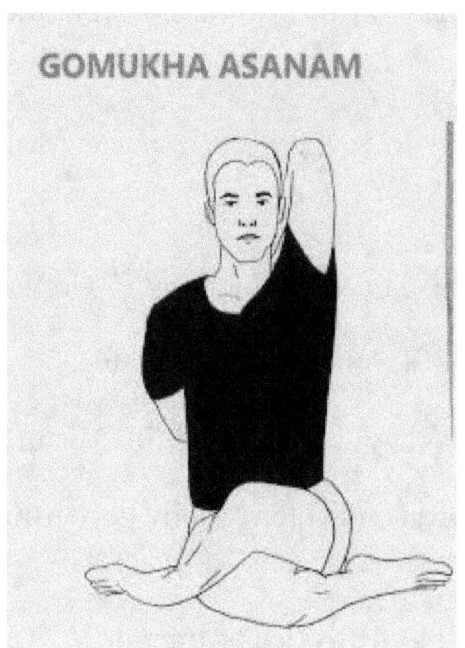

GOMUKHA ASANAM

DEFINATION

Dear reader today am going to illustrate about gomukhaasanam .it is joining of three words first one is go in English meaning it is pointed as cow, mukha means faces, and asanam means posture, so it is called as cow face asanam .in some other text this posture are give meaning as light when performing this posture our face become very bright full it is one of practical experience.

one who wants to do this posture .mainly the person with empty stomach ,and evacuate stools and urine .particularly free bowel movement is mainly presented when doing this posture .Small amount of water may be drink, ,take right place to perform this posture, without any disturbance ,..spread the bed sheet and yoga mate ,and stand with a focused mind with concentration ,take deep breath and exhale do this for at least three to five minutes.

Sit on the mat and stretch the both legs ,first you have to fold the left leg and placed under the right buttocks .

The under the right buttocks.

Then you have to fold the right leg, and kept under the left buttocks,

The right knee placed above the left knee

Then you have to sit erectly, and lift right arm and placed behind the chest in between two schapoid bone

And bend the left arm behind the chest and catch the right palm .in this posture the right elbow should be top on the head region.

Try two maintain this posture for two to three minutes, it very difficulty in initial stage, latter it is possible to make very easy this posture.

BENEFITS

When folding the two legs it will give strengthen to external genital organ and it improve the blood supply,

The haemorrhoids are get reduced due to by profound blood supply to anus.

Uncontrolled urination in females are get reduced by this posture.

The blood passes to different position at a same time, the cardiac muscle get benefitted .if there any blockage it well get reduced by this posture,

It give more concentration than other posture ,in some stone sculpture some sages perform this posture .

It relieve stress and strain.

Arm and shoulder muscle get strengthen.

CONTRAINDICATION

Those who are affected by sciatica ,cervical spondilities are advised to not perform this posture.

And elder with knee problem or other arthritic disorder not advice this posture,

1-Those who are suffered by hip and leg disorder or fracture.

2-During menstrual time.

3-Suffering from liver cirrhosis or stomach ulceration are not advised do this posture.

4-those who are pregnant.

5-any undergone abdominal surgery.

6- Bedridden.

7-after taking heavy meals and empty stomach.

8-before sleep this posture usually not advised .

9-person with any fracture in hand s and dislocation of the shoulder joint not advised to do this posture.

10-without proper sleep and diet you should not perform this posture.

11-befoer going to bed not advised to do this posture.

17-KURMA ASANAM

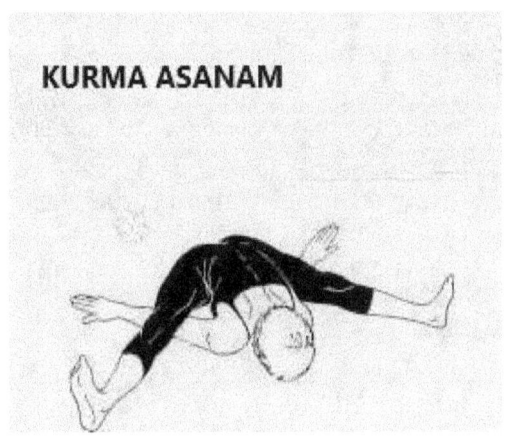

KURMA ASANAM

DEFINATION

The etymology the word meaning of **KURMA** means tortoise and asanam means posture, so the tortoise posture is called as **KURMASASNAM**.one of pancharatra text in vaishnavam samprathayam has mentioned about this asanam .the tortoise is one of living animals more than 200 years ,and it can possible to live in water and earth also .even it can lived in very hot and extreme cold climate also. in emergency condition it inhale its limps and head to its shell ,even ferocious animal also not able to bite it .

Unlike other posture , It is very difficult one, those who wants to do this posture .mainly the person   with empty stomach ,and evacuate stools and urine .particularly free bowel movement is mainly presented when doing this posture .Small amount of water may be drink, ,take right place to perform this posture, without any disturbance ,..spread the bed sheet and yoga mate ,and stand with a focused mind with concentration ,take deep breath and exhale do this for at least three to five minutes.

Sit on the mat in a comfortable position.

Then slowly stretched out the two legs.

The knees are bent slightly; maintain the heels are contact with the earth.

The body is leaned forward from the hips and the hands slid under the knees. The body leans forward (bending at the hips).

Then you have to allow the hands and arms to slide sideways and backward under the knees until the elbows lie near the back of the knees.

The legs are stretched forward and legs are straightened as much as possible. The forehead is brought to touch the mat.

If it possible the arms are further brought around the back to interlock the hands under the buttocks.

Otherwise you can simply stretch the hand outward position only.

Then come to normal posture,

Its very difficult one .before doing this posture you can take some precaution method.

And you should maintain this posture up to two to three minute in advanced states in early states one minute duration is enough.

BENEFITS

_This posture is very much beneficial to internal abdominal organ and respiratory system.

It improved the blood supply to head and neck.

Concentration and memory power get increased by this posture.

This posture is cured the curvature of the spine .and spinal muscle and nerves also get benefited by this posture.

It improves the appetite and relieved the constipation and flatulence.

Stress and strain also cured by this posture.

CONTRAINDICATION

Those who are affected by spinal disorder are advised to not perform this posture.

And elder with knee problem or other arthritic disorder not advice this posture,

1-Those who are suffered by hip and leg disorder or fracture.

2-During menstrual time.

3-Suffering from liver cirrhosis or stomach ulceration are not advised do this posture.

4-those who are pregnant.

5-any undergone abdominal surgery.

6- Bedridden.

7-after taking heavy meals and empty stomach.

8-before sleep this posture usually not advised.

9-person with any fracture in hand s and dislocation of the shoulder joint not advised to do this posture.

10-without proper sleep and diet you should not perform this posture .

11-befoer going to bed not advised to do this posture.

18- SETHUBANDHA SARVANGA ASANAM

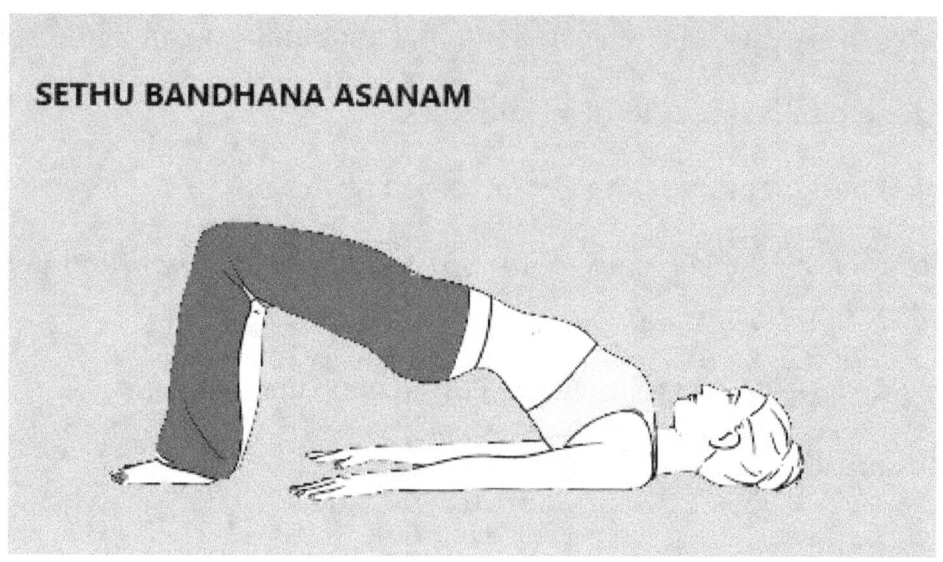

SETHU BANDHANA ASANAM

DEFINATION

Dear reader today am going to illustrate, about **_SETHU BANDHA SARVANGA ASANAM_** it is one of very famous posture in olden days even though children's are doing their in playing time ,the word meaning for SSETHU is bridge and BANDHA means bond and sarvanga means total body has involved this posture and asanam means posture ,so this posture is simply called as bridge posture. Any one does this posture.

One of 19' century book called as SRITATVANIDI has mentioned this posture in the name of KAAMAPITHASANAM .

It is very simple one to do this posture, but some premonitory method and step is needed for all posture. one who wants to do this posture .mainly the person with empty stomach ,and evacuate stools and urine .particularly free bowel movement is mainly presented when doing this posture .Small amount of water may be drink, ,take right place to perform this posture, without any disturbance ,.spread the bed sheet and yoga mate ,and stand with a focused mind with concentration ,take deep breath and exhale do this for at least three to five minutes.

Then lie down on the yoga mat in supine position.

You have to slowly rise the both knee above the ground level .

Then give force and lift the whole body by pressing the both hand on the earth.

Then you have to try catching the heels by the palms and keeping it for at least two minute duration .

And come to normal position slowly some authors are mentioned the keep down and rise the body repeat, but there is no evidence in shastrical literature.

BENEFITS

This posture provides good strength and flexibility to spine muscle and nerves.

whole body get refreshed by this posture,

It reduced the flatulence .

It improved the blood circulation all over the body.

Vision power of eye gets improved by this posture.

CONTRAINDICATION

Those who are affected by spine disorder are advised to not perform this posture.

And elder with knee problem or other arthritic disorder not advice this posture,.

1-Those who are suffered by hip and leg disorder or fracture.

2-During menstrual time.

3-Suffering from liver cirrhosis or stomach ulceration are not advised do this posture.

4-those who are pregnant.

5-any undergone abdominal surgery.

6- Bedridden.

7-after taking heavy meals and empty stomach.

8-before sleep this posture usually not advised .

9-person with any fracture in hand s and dislocation of the shoulder joint not advised to do this posture.

10-without proper sleep and diet you should not perform this posture .

11-befoer going to bed not advised to do this posture.

19- MATSYASANAM

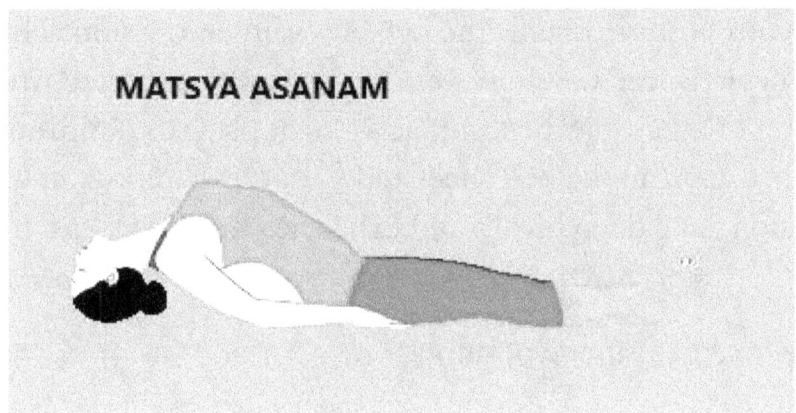

MATSYA ASANAM

DEFINATION

Dear reader today am going to illustrate about MATSYAASANAM one of the ancient literature has GHERANTA SAMHITHA has described this posture the word meaning for matshya is fish and the word asanam means posture so, the fish posture is called as matsya asanam.

Some authors correlate this posture relevant to lord *VISHNU* because he take fish avadar [form]to product this earth from anti god peoples in hatha yoga pradipika this posture is counter opposite to sarvanga posture .but whatever it may be the posture resembled like fish is called as *MATSYAASANAM* .

one who wants to do this posture .mainly the person   with empty stomach ,and evacuate stools and urine .particularly free bowel movement is mainly presented when doing this posture .Small amount of water may be drink, ,take right place to perform this posture, without any disturbance ,.spread the bed sheet and yoga mate ,and stand with a focused mind with concentration ,take deep breath and exhale do this for at least three to five minutes.

Lie down on the yoga mat in a supine position,

First you have lift the right leg and fold kept near to inguinal region of the thigh .

Now you can fold the right leg and kept in left inguinal area .

Should note that both legs are in crossed section .now you have catch left toe with right palm,

And right toe with left palm .

Now breathe deeply then lift the chest by placing the head in downward position,

Keep it for two minute duration then come to normal position,

BENEFITS

This posture is good for those who suffered by respiratory disorder .

The meditation power will get improved by this posture.

The memory and concentration power will improved by this posture so, this posture is very beneficial for school students,

It increases the production of gastric juice and bile juice our appetites will increases and the digestion capacity will increase.

Tones the abdominal walls and thighs .

This posture provide strength to chest muscle .

The holding capacity of air in lungs gets increased.

The children's those who are affected by asthma they very soon get relief from this posture.

The abdominal wall get tightened, so, this asana prevent the herniation disorder.

The stress and strain are get relieved by this posture.

CONTRAINDICATION

Those who are affected by vertebral disorder are advised to not perform this posture.

And elder with knee problem or other arthritic disorder not advice this posture,

1-Those who are suffered by hip and leg disorder or fracture.

2-During menstrual time.

3-Suffering from liver cirrhosis or stomach ulceration are not advised do this posture.

4-those who are pregnant.

5-any undergone abdominal surgery.

6- Bedridden.

7-after taking heavy meals and empty stomach.

8-before sleep this posture usually not advised.

9-person with any fracture in hand s and dislocation of the shoulder joint not advised to do this posture.

10-without proper sleep and diet you should not perform this posture .

11-befoer going to bed not advised to do this posture.

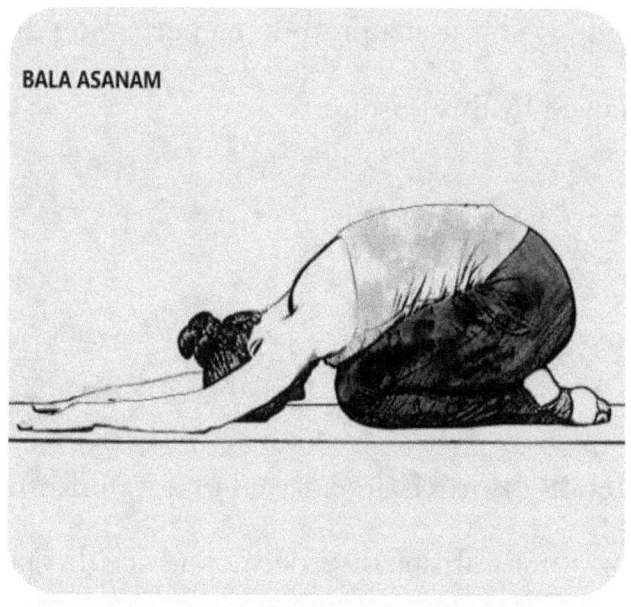

BALA ASANAM

DEFINATION

Dear reader today am going to illustrate about BALASANAM .the word meaning for bala is child and asanam means posture so this posture is called as child posture .one of the 19' century book *SRITATVANIDI* is mentioned this posture as **KANDUKAASANAM** some of modern authors are mentioned this posture .when a toddler is getting rest like this posture so it is called as *BALASANASM.*

Among other posture it is one very simple and best one every one during their young age they should perform this posture in their child hood .one who wants to do this posture .mainly the person with empty stomach ,and evacuate stools and urine .particularly free bowel movement is mainly presented when doing this posture .Small amount of water may be drink, ,take right place to perform this posture, without any disturbance ,.spread the bed sheet and yoga mate ,and stand with a focused mind with concentration ,take deep breath and exhale do this for at least three to five minutes.

First you have to Kneel down on the yoga mat and you sit on your heels with comfortable position

Bend forward, and touch the mat by forehead.

And place the arm on the mat with stretched out from the body . and palm is in prone position.

Then maintain the posture up to five minute duration meanwhile this time you have to breath wave .not forced one.

While doing this posture is provide good sleep during this posture is good indication of this posture .

Then slowly come to normal position.

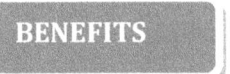

BENEFITS

Reduced the stress and strain feel like young child.

Before going to bed this posture is recommended.

blood supply to the brain has improved by this posture.

Those who are affected by cardiac asthma this posture give very much support to them .but necessary precaution is taken.

Flatulence get removed by this posture.

The memory and concentration power will improved by this posture so, this posture is very beneficial for school students,

Stress and strain also cured by this posture.

CONTRAINDICATION

And elder with knee problem or other arthritic disorder not advice this posture,

1-Those who are suffered by hip and leg disorder or fracture.

2-During menstrual time.

3-Suffering from liver cirrhosis or stomach ulceration are not advised do this posture.

4-those who are pregnant.

5-any undergone abdominal surgery.

6- Bedridden.

7-after taking heavy meals and empty stomach.

8-before sleep this posture usually not advised .

9-person with any fracture in hand s and dislocation of the shoulder joint not advised to do this posture.

10-without proper sleep and diet you should not perform this posture.

11-befoer going to bed not advised to do this posture.

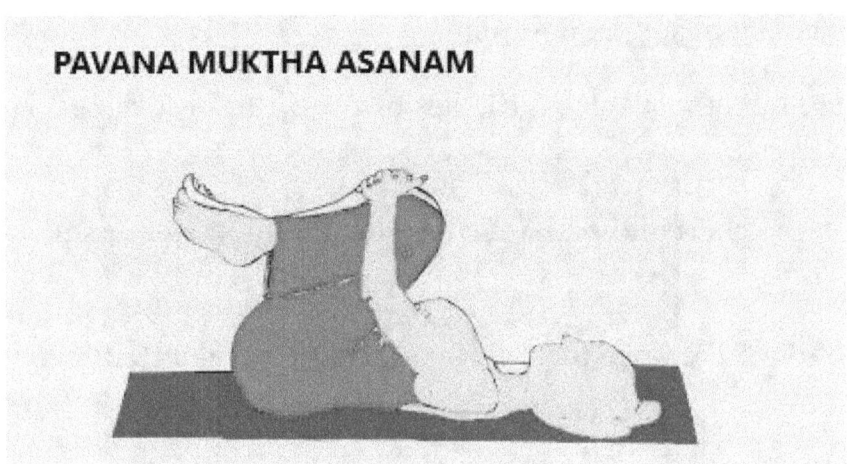

PAVANA MUKTHA ASANAM

DEFINATION

Dear reader today am going to illustrate about *PAVANAMUTAASANAM*.it has joining of three word ,in Sanskrit the word *PAVANAM means wind and MUKTHA means relieving or attain moksham* and asanam means posture .so it is called as air relieving posture from our body is called as PAVANAMUTHAASANAM .

flatulent is one of the waste product in form of air ,it usually during the digestive process .when large amount of the gas deposit in our body will lead to produced various disorder like pain ,excessive flatulence .pricking pain all over the body loss of appetite ,anorexia ,are produced in mild nature ,when they are very sever they lead to neurological disorder like paralysis etc are produced by the flatulence .this flatulence is also called in ayurveda is atho vayu .further you Want know about vata and theory you have to refer in *AYURVEDA KOSTA TO SAKA THEORY* .

PROCEDURE

This one of very simple posture even children's to elder people can perform this posture. But basic premonitory effort should be taken is needed for all types of posture is essential. one who wants to do this posture .mainly the person with empty stomach ,and evacuate stools and urine .particularly free bowel movement is mainly presented when doing this posture .Small amount of water may be drink, ,take right place to perform this posture, without any disturbance ,.spread the bed sheet and yoga mate ,and stand with a focused mind with concentration ,take deep breath and exhale do this for at least three to five minutes.

Then you have toile down on the yoga mat in supine position.

Then slowly raise the knee and folded then the two leg is catches by two palm by locking posture.

Then slowly placed the both knee on the chest and pressure given to abdomen by presses their abdomen with their left leg.

Meanwhile time your chin is tried to touch the knee then only you have to produce enough pressure to the abdomen.

then he presses abdomen with both legs, placing their chin between their knees. From this position, the yogi swings their body back and forth 5 to 10 times,

During this posture some amount of gases is passed out but, don't give extreme pressure to abdomen.

Then come back to normal posture.

BENEFITS

This posture removed the flatulence from the body .

Staged faeces are passed out from the body .

Improve the appetite and digestion.

This posture produced light feeling to the body .

Heaviness in the abdomen and chest are reduced by this posture.

This posture is proven posture, it provide strength to external genital organs.

It released the constipation and flatulence,

Sciatica and degeneration of the lumbar and sacral nerve are get cured by this posture,

The forearms and arms are get strengthened by this posture.

Reduce the belly fat and tighten the abdominal wall and prevent the herniation disorder.

This posture has provide good appetite .

Uterine problem will also get subsided by this posture.

CONTRAINDICATION

Those who are affected by sciatica, cervical spondilities are advised to not perform this posture.

And elder with knee problem or other arthritic disorder not advice this posture,.

1-Those who are suffered by hip and leg disorder or fracture.

2-During menstrual time.

3-Suffering from liver cirrhosis or stomach ulceration are not advised do this posture.

4-those who are pregnant.

5-any undergone abdominal surgery.

6- Bedridden.

7-after taking heavy meals and empty stomach.

8-before sleep this posture usually not advised.

9-person with any fracture in hand s and dislocation of the shoulder joint not advised to do this posture.

10-without proper sleep and diet you should not perform this posture.

11-befoer going to bed not advised to do this posture.

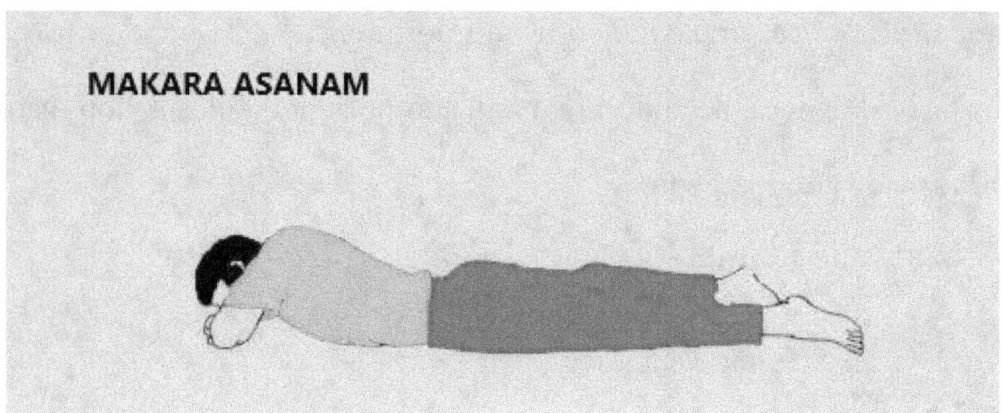

MAKARA ASANAM

Dear reader today am going to illustrate about **MAKARASANAM** the word meaning **MAKARA** is denote to astrological term is **CAPRICORN** constellation .its symbol is goat in take rest position .BUT here the **WORD MEANING FOR MAKARAM** means crocodile its living in water and earth and it's the animal vehicle of lord **VARUNA** and **GANGA** matha .and asanam means posture so the crocodile posture is called as **MAKARASANAM.**

One of the seventeenth century text ***GHRENDA samhitha*** has described about this posture.

one who wants to do this posture .mainly the person   with empty stomach ,and evacuate stools and urine .particularly free bowel movement is mainly presented when doing this posture .Small amount of water may be drink, ,take right place to perform this posture, without any disturbance ,..spread the bed sheet and yoga mate ,and stand with a focused mind with concentration ,take deep breath and exhale do this for at least three to five minutes.

Simply lie down on the yoga mat in prone posture .

Stretched out the leg in outwards direction and sure that the body is not movable.

The two arms are crossed and kept under the head .

Make sure that your fore head is rest on the wrist of the hand .

Then keep it for at least three to five minute duration meanwhile time you may get sleep no need to worry about the sleep.

Then slowly come to normal posture by removing the hand side wards to the body.

Some authors tell to lift the head like opening of the crocodile mouth .but it is not mentioned the text.

BENEFITS

This posture is very much beneficial to the head and neck.

Cervical spondilities are get relieved by this posture.

The person affected by insomnia this posture is very much helpful to them.

It one of the relaxing posture and support the body from stress and strain.

This posture is very much beneficial to respiratory system. And asthma also gets relieved by this posture.

It improved the blood supply to head and neck.

Concentration and memory power get increased by this posture.

This posture is cured the curvature of the spine .and spinal muscle and nerves also get benefited by this posture.

It improves the appetite and relived the constipation and flatulence.

Stress and strain also cured by this posture.

CONTRAINDICATION

Those who are affected by sciatica, cervical spondilities are advised to not perform this posture.

And elder with knee problem or other arthritic disorder not advice this posture,.

1-Those who are suffered by hip and leg disorder or fracture.

2-During menstrual time.

3-Suffering from liver cirrhosis or stomach ulceration are not advised do this posture.

4-those who are pregnant.

5-any undergone abdominal surgery.

6- Bedridden.

7-after taking heavy meals and empty stomach.

8-before sleep this posture usually not advised .

9-person with any fracture in hand s and dislocation of the shoulder joint not advised to do this posture.

10-without proper sleep and diet you should not perform this posture.

 11-befoer going to bed not advised to do this posture.

23-SAVASANAM

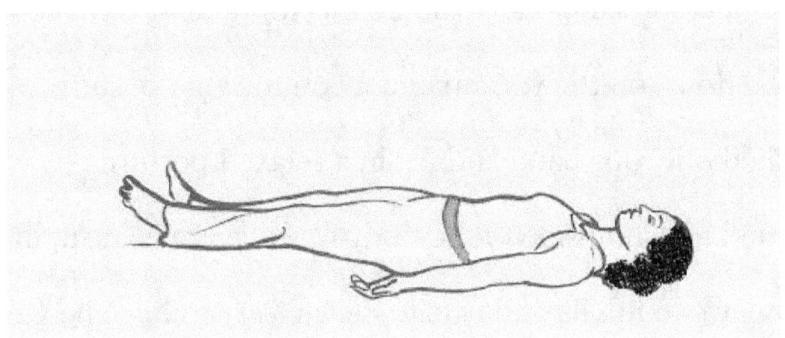

DEFINATION

Dear reader today am going to illustrate about SAVASANAM normally it 's joining of two letter one is sava and another one is asanam ,the sava mean corpse or dead body ,and asasnam means posture ,the posture resemble like corpse is called as savasasnasm .nobody knows about what is held inside of the corpse ,so here we give the word resemble like .the corpse is absence of breath but here breath only take place .that like peace and calm produced by the posture .

One of the fifteenth century book *hathayoga pradeepika* had illustrated about this posture, this posture is reduced all complication of other posture, so it should be performed after other posture are performed.

PROCEDURE

This one of very easiest one every one can performed this posture ,those who wants to do this posture .mainly the person with empty stomach ,and evacuate stools and urine .particularly free bowel movement is mainly presented when doing this posture .Small amount of water may be drink, ,take right place to perform this posture, without any disturbance ,.spread the bed sheet and yoga mate ,and stand with a focused mind with concentration ,take deep breath and exhale do this for at least three to five minutes.

Then you should lie down on the yoga mat in a comfortable posture.

You have to stretched out your hand and leg in a relaxed posture .

The hand is extended to lateral side of the body m the palm is in supine position.

In this posture you have to inhale and exhale the air very mildly and calm mind .

This posture lead to good sleep you don't bother about it.

And try to maintain up to 15-20 minute duration, then you come to normal posture.

Then you have to practice pranayama then come to normal posture.

BENEFITS

Unlike other posture this posture create good calm and peaceful to the mind.

This posture is rejuvenating the body and minds.

Memory power and concentration has improved by this posture.

Body stress and strain are getting relieved by this posture.

Blood supply to all organ's are uniformly supplied.

This posture provide refreshment to whole day without any doubt,

Mental intolerance are balanced by this posture.

CONTRAINDICATION

1-Those who are suffered by hip and leg disorder or fracture.

2-During menstrual time.

3-Suffering from liver cirrhosis or stomach ulceration are not advised do this posture.

4-those who are pregnant.

5-any undergone abdominal surgery.

6- Bedridden.

7-after taking heavy meals and empty stomach.

8-before sleep this posture usually not advised .

9-person with any fracture in hand s and dislocation of the shoulder joint not advised to do this posture.

10-without proper sleep and diet you should not perform this posture.

11-befoer going to bed not advised to do this posture.

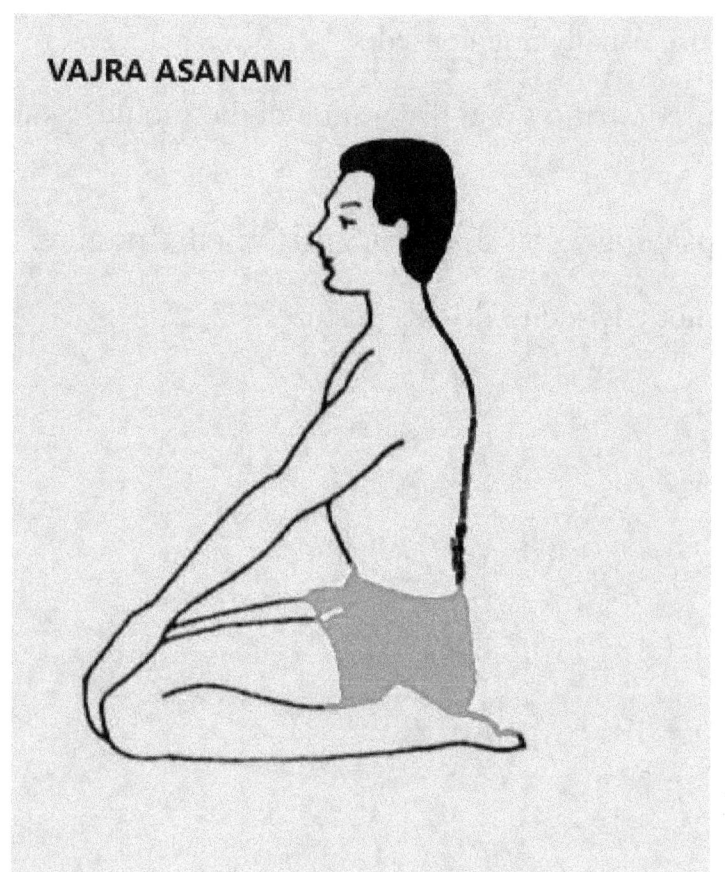

VAJRA ASANAM

DEFINATION

Dear reader today am going to illustrate about **VAJRASANAM,** one of the fifteenth century literature ***HATHAYOGA PRADHEEPIKA*** has described this posture as sidhasanam, normally the word meaning VAJRA IS an instrument or thunder bold or diamond is called as vajram above the meaning we come to one understand is some this is hard or powerful is called as vajram and asanam means posture so the diamond posture is called as *vajrasanam* .

But in yoga mimamsa dharsan the **VAJRAM** means weapon and *GHERANDA samhitha* also described this posture .in modern days some authors give some sub types and other name but thre is literature evidence for their view.

PROCEDURE

one who wants to do this posture .mainly the person   with empty stomach ,and evacuate stools and urine .particularly free bowel movement is mainly presented when doing this posture .Small amount of water may be drink, ,take right place to perform this posture, without any disturbance ,.spread the bed sheet and yoga mate ,and stand with a focused mind with concentration ,take deep breath and exhale do this for at least three to five minutes.

Slowly sit on the yoga mat in a knee down posture their buttocks is placed on the both heels .The two toes are placed on the earth in a erect posture, basically the total weight is supported by two toes only.

Then you have sit in a erect .posture.

Keep it up for at least two minute and come to normal posture,.

While come to normal posture should slowly come to normal posture or it will lead to some pain in the toes.

BENEFITS

Lower limp are get nourished by this posture .and this posture improve the blood supply to the lower limp.

Concentration power get improved by this posture.

This posture improves the digestive power .and appetite will increased.

It removes the flatulence in the lower abdomen.

The spine is erect in while doing this posture so it is very useful in meditation purpose.

Some modern orthopaedic surgeon are not recommended this posture , because while doing this posture it will create some orthopaedic problem .but our strong recommendation without proper training you don't do any posture ,.

And elder with knee problem or other arthritic disorder not advice this posture.,

1-Those who are suffered by hip and leg disorder or fracture.

2-During menstrual time.

3-Suffering from liver cirrhosis or stomach ulceration are not advised do this posture.

4-those who are pregnant.

5-any undergone abdominal surgery.

6- Bedridden.

7-after taking heavy meals and empty stomach

.8-before sleep this posture usually not advised.

9-person with any fracture in hand s and dislocation of the shoulder joint not advised to do this posture.

10-without proper sleep and diet you should not perform this posture .

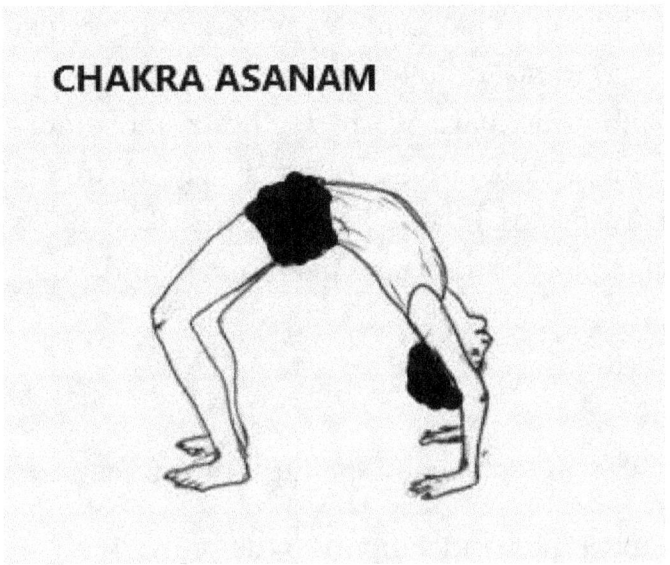

CHAKRA ASANAM

DEFINATION

Dear reader today am going to illustrate about CHAKRA ASANAM ,it is joining of two words one is CHAKRAM and other one is asanam ,the chakra has denotes to the word meaning of wheel and asanam means posture ,so the wheel like posture is called as chakra asanam .this posture now a day's performed in the gymnastics and circus in modern days but today the people do this posture for they getting ability to bend their body in backward position but this posture is mentioned in Vedic days as have the therapeutic importance ,.

There are artha chakra asanam and kati chakra asanam are some sub types in this posture, but here i have mentioned only normal chakra asanam every one can perform this posture as their regular practice of the yoga procedure.

For beginners it is very difficult to perform this posture but regular practice of this posture make it easy ,so ,one who wants to do this posture .mainly the person with empty stomach ,and evacuate stools and urine .particularly free bowel movement is mainly presented when doing this posture .Small amount of water may be drink, ,take right place to perform this posture, without any disturbance ,..spread the bed sheet and yoga mate ,and stand with a focused mind with concentration ,take deep breath and exhale do this for at least three to five minutes.

Stand erectly on the yoga mat.

Then you have to pace your palm on the back of the hip near upper parts of the buttocks.

Slowly bend backwards by keeping the hand support to the body,

Then the body come to middle level then you have to place the hand on the earth

Make the body backward bend, like arch.

Then keep it for two minutes duration.

And keep the one hand support on the earth move another hand to lift the body to come to normal posture.

Then keep standing in normal posture.

It's get some difficulty while doing this posture initially but regular practice make it perfect.

BENEFITS

This posture is very helpful to reduce the hyper tension.

Internal abdominal organs are functioning well.

It improve the digestive function,

The sexual function gets improved by this posture.

This posture will stimulate the liver secretion and increase the appetite and flatulence.

Reduce the abdominal fat and abdominal muscles are getting strengthened by this posture.

Spine muscle and back muscle get strengthened by this posture.

This posture is very much beneficial to the head and neck.

Cervical spondilities are get relieved by this posture.

The person affected by insomnia this posture is very much helpful to them.

It one of the relaxing posture and support the body from stress and strain.

This posture is very much beneficial to respiratory system. And asthma also gets relieved by this posture.

It improved the blood supply to head and neck.

CONTRAINDICATION

Those who are affected by sciatica, cervical spondilities are advised to not perform this posture.

And elder with knee problem or other arthritic disorder not advice this posture,

Those who affected by vertigo positional vertigo and giddiness are not advice do this posture.

1-Those who are suffered by hip and leg disorder or fracture.

2-During menstrual time.

3-Suffering from liver cirrhosis or stomach ulceration are not advised do this posture

4-those who are pregnant.

5-any undergone abdominal surgery.

6- Bedridden.

7-after taking heavy meals and empty stomach.

8-before sleep this posture usually not advised.

9-person with any fracture in hand s and dislocation of the shoulder joint not advised to do this posture.

10-without proper sleep and diet you should not perform this posture.

11-befoer going to bed not advised to do this posture.

26-HALASANAM

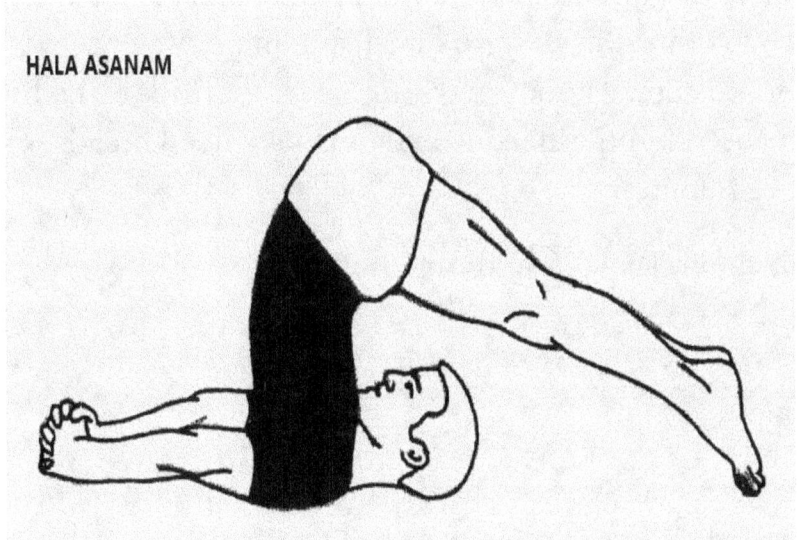

HALA ASANAM

Dear reader today am going to illustrate about **HALASANAM** one of the nineteenth century literature sritatvanidhi has illustrated about this posture ,it one of the difficult posture, by practice this posture is easier than other posture .thre are two words joining and produced the halasanam word .the first one meaning is plough for the word HALA ,and asanam means posture ,the plough posture is called as halasanam ,in olden days the farmer doing agriculture with the help of plough they ploughing the soil for agriculture likewise this posture is helpful us to processing our mind for yoga .

the definition i indicate that ,this posture is somewhat difficult to perform this posture .so take premonitory step is essential for this posture, those, who wants to do this posture .mainly the person with empty stomach ,and evacuate stools and urine .particularly free bowel movement is mainly presented when doing this posture .Small amount of water may be drink, ,take right place to perform this posture, without any disturbance ,.spread the bed sheet and yoga mate ,and stand with a focused mind with concentration ,take deep breath and exhale do this for at least three to five minutes.

Lie on the yoga mat in a supine position, and relax your body and mind.

Then you have to lift your legs.

Then you put the hand to support the hip region.

Slowly raise the hips to and the thigh is placed above the chest level .then your two foot are placed on the earth level and maintain the posture up to two minutes .then come to normal stage slowly .

{Your hand is stretched out direct position on the earth level only}.

BENEFITS

This posture is best for reducing the weight loss, it reduced the abdominal fat ,and tighten the abdominal wall.

It reduced the flatulence and improves the appetites.

it stimulate the internal abdominal organ and normalised the secretion .

it reduced the stress and strain .

The menses problem and PCO disorder are get relieved by this posture

And regulate the menstrual cycle ,.

It stimulate the external sex organs .

CONTRAINDICATION

Those who are affected by sciatica ,cervical spondilities are advised to not perform this posture.

And elder with knee problem or other arthritic disorder not advice this posture,.

1-Those who are suffered by hip and leg disorder or fracture.

2-During menstrual time.

3-Suffering from liver cirrhosis or stomach ulceration are not advised do this posture.

4-those who are pregnant.

5-any undergone abdominal surgery.

6- Bedridden.

7-after taking heavy meals and empty stomach.

8-before sleep this posture usually not advised .

9-person with any fracture in hand s and dislocation of the shoulder joint not advised to do this posture.

10-without proper sleep and diet you should not perform this posture .

11-befoer going to bed not advised to do this posture.

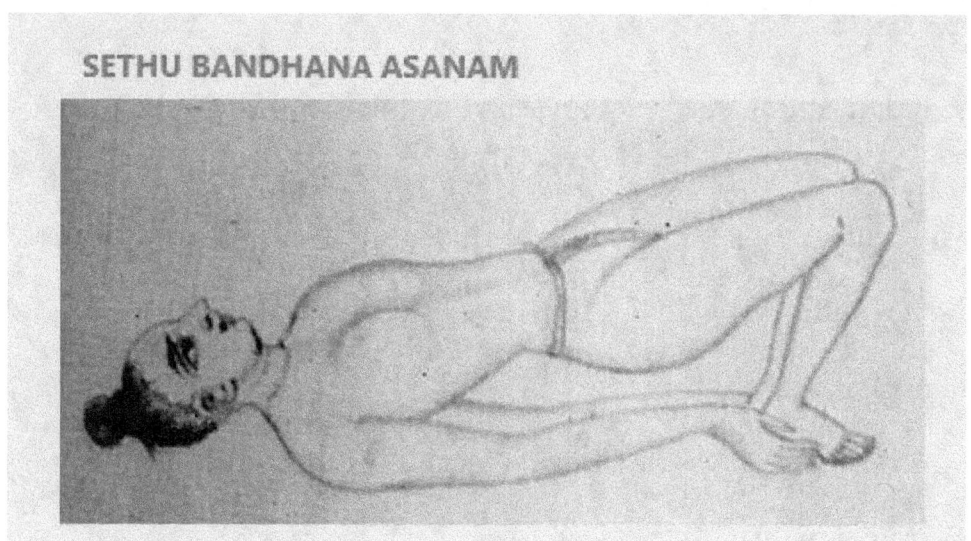

SETHU BANDHANA ASANAM

DEFINATION

Dear reader today am going to illustrate about **SETHUBANDHANA ASANAM** or this posture is called as **SETHUBANDHANA SARVANGA ASASNAM**, The total organ are involved in this posture so this posture is called as sethubandha sarvanga asanam .one of the nineteenth century book *srithathvanithi* has illustrated this posture as **KAMAPITHA ASANAM** .

The word meaning for sethu is belongs to bridge ,and bandha means bond or attachment or in simple term is called as catch .and asanam means posture .so bridge like posture is called as sethubandha asanam .make the body like bridge ,with the help of hand by catch the heel make it this structure .

It's one of the easiest posture to perform ,but maintain this posture some extended time is very difficult ,so proper practice is needed for this posture .those , who wants to do this posture .mainly the person   with empty stomach ,and evacuate stools and urine .particularly free bowel movement is mainly presented when doing this posture .Small amount of water may be drink, ,take right place to perform this posture, without any disturbance ,.spread the bed sheet and yoga mate ,and stand with a focused mind with concentration ,take deep breath and exhale do this for at least three to five minutes.

Lie down on the yoga mat in supine posture.

Place the palm face on the earth.

Then you have to fold the knee, and the heel is catches by the hand .

Now you have to lift the body by given the pressure by head and neck.

Your head and neck only placed on the earth,

Some authors indicate that to lift the body up and down simultaneously but here it is not recommended because the aim of the yoga is to produce calm to mind and body.

Then you have to come normal posture.

BENEFITS

This posture provides good strength to neck and chest muscle.

The lung capacity is increased and reduce the respiratory disorder .

This posture provides calm to mind and relieve the stress and strain.

 Provide good appetite.

Reduced the abdominal fat.

Reduce the uterine disorder .and menstrual cramps.

It stimulate the external sex organs

This posture produced light feeling to the body

Heaviness in the abdomen and chest are reduced by this posture

This posture is proven posture, it provide strength to external genital organs.

It released the constipation and flatulence,

CONTRAINDICATION

Those who are affected by sciatica, cervical spondilities are advised to not perform this posture.

And elder with knee problem or other arthritic disorder not advice this posture,

1-Those who are suffered by hip and leg disorder or fracture.

2-During menstrual time.

3-Suffering from liver cirrhosis or stomach ulceration are not advised do this posture.

4-those who are pregnant.

5-any undergone abdominal surgery.

6- Bedridden.

7-after taking heavy meals and empty stomach.

8-before sleep this posture usually not advised.

9-person with any fracture in hand s and dislocation of the shoulder joint not advised to do this posture.

10-without proper sleep and diet you should not perform this posture.

11-befoer going to bed not advised to do this posture.

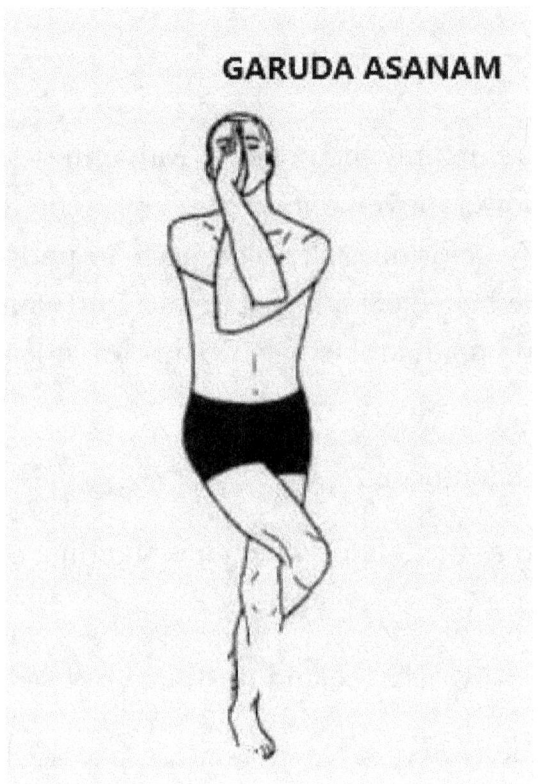

GARUDA ASANAM

Dear reader today am going to illustrate about *GARUDAASANAM*,the word garuda is indicate the divine bird EAGLE of lord Vishnu ,in hidhu mythology lord Vishnu has get very important roll to product the universe and product he people from various disorder and disaster .and the divine bird garuda is having very powerful bird ,it destruction all enemy likewise the this posture product the people from various disease and disorder .this posture is asymmetrical posture but it get very important role in the yogig science .

One of the seventeenth century book *GHERANDA SAMHITHA* has mentioned this posture .and nineteenth century book srithathvanithi has illustrated about this posture.

one who wants to do this posture .mainly the person with empty stomach ,and evacuate stools and urine .particularly free bowel movement is mainly presented when doing this posture .Small amount of water may be drink, ,take right place to perform this posture, without any disturbance ,.spread the bed sheet and yoga mate ,and stand with a focused mind with concentration ,take deep breath and exhale do this for at least three to five minutes.

Standing on the yoga mat in a mountain pose .

Take the right leg forward direction to the left leg which it is standing on the earth, and put the right above the heel on the left leg .

{Note the right leg should be catches by right toe and next finger of right toe}

Then you have to slightly bend the left leg .

Now you have to stretched out your hands and make it cross the right palm should be placed on the left hand for arm lateral posture, like two snake mating and keep it for two to three minute and come to normal posture .

This posture is mainly balance our body .the balance coordination function is mainly related to neuromuscular proper function.

Concentration and memory power will increased by this posture.

Vision power gets improved by this posture.

It strength the lower limp .and flexibility get increased by this posture,

It relieved the flatulence and staged tools .and increase the appetite.

heaviness in the abdomen and chest are reduced by this posture.

This posture is proven posture, it provide strength to external genital organs.

Those who are affected by sciatica, cervical spondilities are advised to not perform this posture.

And elder with knee problem or other arthritic disorder not advice this posture,

1-Those who are suffered by hip and leg disorder or fracture.

2-During menstrual time.

3-Suffering from liver cirrhosis or stomach ulceration are not advised do this posture.

4-those who are pregnant.

5-any undergone abdominal surgery.

6- Bedridden.

7-after taking heavy meals and empty stomach.

8-before sleep this posture usually not advised .

9-person with any fracture in hand s and dislocation of the shoulder joint not advised to do this posture.

10-without proper sleep and diet you should not perform this posture.

11-befoer going to bed not advised to do this posture.

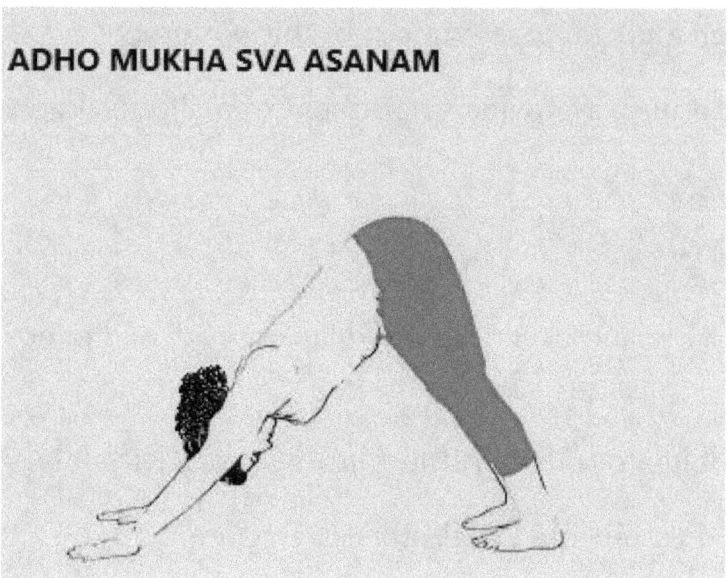

ADHO MUKHA SVA ASANAM

DEFINATION

Dear reader today am going to illustrate about ADHOMUKASVA ASANAM, this one of the very familiar asasnam in ancient yoga culture .one of the eighteen century yoga literature *HATHABHYASAPATHATHI* has illustrated this posture in the name of gajaasanam ,but some authors are give opinion that this posture is not similar one ,.

The word meaning ADHO means downward and MUKHA means face and the word SVA means dog and asanam means posture .so the face of the dog in downward face position is called as adho mukha sva asanam.

This one of the normal posture not so much difficulty so those , who wants to do this posture .mainly the person with empty stomach ,and evacuate stools and urine .particularly free bowel movement is mainly presented when doing this posture .Small amount of water may be drink, ,take right place to perform this posture, without any disturbance ,.spread the bed sheet and yoga mate ,and stand with a focused mind with concentration ,take deep breath and exhale do this for at least three to five minutes.

Then you have lie down on the yoga mat in a prone posture,.

Then you have to lift the body by given force by the arm,.

Then simultaneously lift the hip by given force on the earth by the two legs.

Make your body like triangular shape, the hip is on the top of your body .and the head is down ward in between two hands .

Now you have look your face upward position and extend the tongue as much as possible and inhale the air and exhale it.

Keep it for two to three minute duration .then come to normal posture.

BENEFITS

The dog having the properties of reduce the body heat naturally like that this posture has the property to reduce the body temperature,.

This posture will help to us balancing our body and mind, and relieving the stress and strain from us.

This posture will reduce the asthma and cardiac asthma also and help to reduce the hypertension.

This posture help to us the brings the abdominal gas in to rectal area and relieve it from the body.

The lung capacity is increased and reduces the respiratory disorder

This posture reduces the menstrual disorder so women can easily perform this posture.

It improved the blood supply to head and neck.

Concentration and memory power get increased by this posture.

This posture is cured the curvature of the spine .and spinal muscle and nerves also get benefited by this posture.

It improves the appetite and relived the constipation and flatulence.

CONTRAINDICATION

Those who are affected by sciatica ,cervical spondilities are advised to not perform this posture.

And elder with knee problem or other arthritic disorder not advice this posture.

1-Those who are suffered by hip and leg disorder or fracture.

2-During menstrual time.

3-Suffering from liver cirrhosis or stomach ulceration are not advised do this posture.

4-those who are pregnant.

5-any undergone abdominal surgery.

6- Bedridden.

7-after taking heavy meals and empty stomach.

8-before sleep this posture usually not advised.

9-person with any fracture in hand s and dislocation of the shoulder joint not advised to do this posture.

10-without proper sleep and diet you should not perform this posture.

11-befoer going to bed not advised to do this posture.

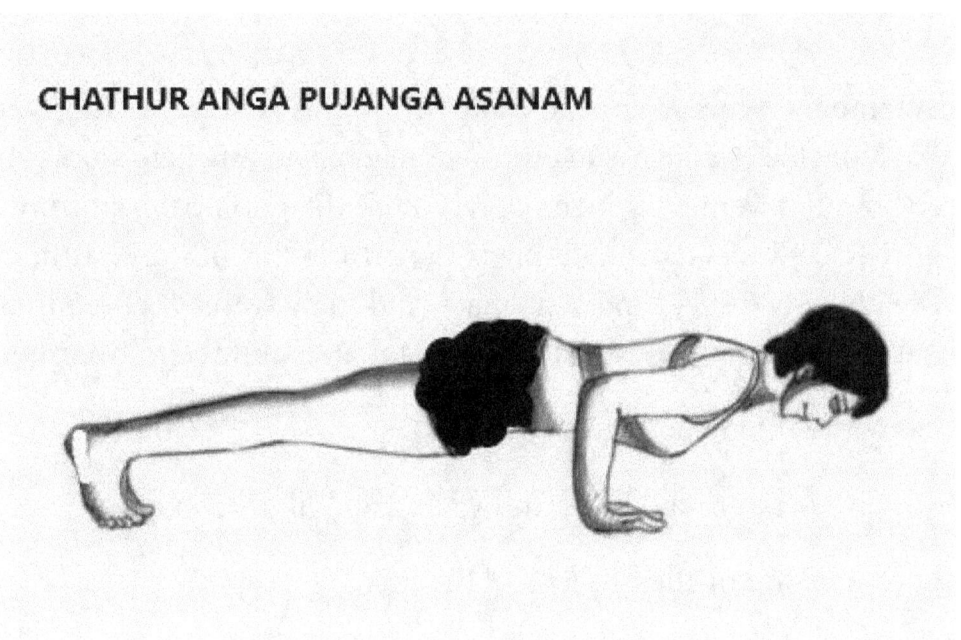

CHATHUR ANGA PUJANGA ASANAM

DEFINATION

Dear reader today am going to illustrate about *CHATHRANGA ASANAM* this posture is otherwise called as CHATHURANGA DANDA ASANAM, this pose has not mentioned in earlier literature but one of the eighteen century book *VYAYAMA DIPIKA* is one of the book has illustrated about physical exercise has illustrated this posture as physical exercise but some authors are mentioned this pose as one of the yoga pose .

The word meaning of CHATHUR means four and ANGA means limps and asanam means posture so four limp has involved in this posture is called as chathuranga asanam.

This one of very simple posture every one can perform this posture so those , who wants to do this posture .mainly the person   with empty stomach ,and evacuate stools and urine .particularly free bowel movement is mainly presented when doing this posture .Small amount of water may be drink, ,take right place to perform this posture, without any disturbance ,.spread the bed sheet and yoga mate ,and stand with a focused mind with concentration ,take deep breath and exhale do this for at least three to five minutes.

Lie one the yoga mat in supine posture .

Then you have to give pressure on the earth by hand and lift the body,

Now you have give pressure by the two toes of the legs.

Your body lift by hand and legs only and not touch the body on the earth.

Keep it for one minute and slowly down the body on the earth by exhaling the air.

And inhale the air and uplift the body again by above mentioned method

Likewise 20 to 25 times you have to perform this posture.

This posture give strength to upper and lower limp.

It reduced the abdominal fat and tightens the abdominal.

The chest muscle get strengthen by this posture .and lung capacity get increased by this posture.

This posture is very much beneficial to respiratory system. And asthma also gets relieved by this posture.

It improved the blood supply to head and neck.

Concentration and memory power get increased by this posture.

This posture is cured the curvature of the spine .and spinal muscle and nerves also get benefited by this posture.

It improves the appetite and relived the constipation and flatulence.

Stress and strain also cured by this posture.

CONTRAINDICATION

Those who are affected by sciatica ,cervical spondilities are advised to not perform this posture.

And elder with knee problem or other arthritic disorder not advice this posture,.

1-Those who are suffered by hip and leg disorder or fracture.

2-During menstrual time.

3-Suffering from liver cirrhosis or stomach ulceration are not advised do this posture.

4-those who are pregnant.

5-any undergone abdominal surgery.

6- Bedridden.

7-after taking heavy meals and empty stomach.

8-before sleep this posture usually not advised .

9-person with any fracture in hand s and dislocation of the shoulder joint not advised to do this posture.

10-without proper sleep and diet you should not perform this posture.

11-befoer going to bed not advised to do this posture.

DEFINATION

[DUE TO DIVINE AND RELEGIOUS REASON WE NOT ADD THE PHOTO HERE READER, KINDLY VISIT THE WEPSITE FOR FURTHER INFORMATION}

Dear reader today am going to illustrate about NATARAJA ASANAM is one of the great pose has practiced in yoga as well as BHARATHA NAATIYAM field ,this one of the classical dance has performed by the GOD SANKARA ,this dance is a cosmic dance has performed with four hands and three eyes on the top of demon's muyalakan.

The word meaning of NATA is come from Tamil language NATANAM and RAJA means kings and asanam means posture .when LORD SIVA performed this dance at the end of the dance he stand this posture ,so final posture is may peak of all performance in the dance so this posture is called KING of the NATANAM pose is called as NATARAJA ASANAM .

LORD SIVA has performed dance in various situation in various place ,in CHIDAMPARAM is place situated in KADALURE district in Tamilnadu. he place competition dance in between THILLAI KALLI at end of the stage he lift the leg and earring the ornament and rotate the body ,during this posture his genital organs are visible .

In THIRUVALANGADU is one of the place near to *THIRUVALLUR DISTRICT*, he performed happy dance with his wife parvathi devi to give moksham to KARAIKAL AMMAIYAR .hear this pose is happy pose but the place is in burial ground .

In MADURAI he performed happy dance but he changed the leg position so it get very important and called as VELLIAMBALAM that means silver dancing place .

The sidhar PATHANJALI has very much interested in seeing the dance at CHIDAMPARAM so here we give the exact posture were the posture is performed in CHIDAMPARAM is called as NATARAJA ASANAM.

Even though this posture is not mentioned in ancient classical text, only modern authors are illustrated various dance posture is not correct .in my view the dance posture is place in Chidambaram only Is correct one,.

It is comes under dancing stage in BARATHA NATIYAM. so ,in olden days they not include under yoga posture ,because now a days the dance Is done for hoppy and enjoyment purpose, but barathanatiyam is differ from modern view it consider as great YOGA POSTURE.

This yogig dance is otherwise called as COSMIC DANCE, it only the divine creature, create the UNIVERSE so, the Indian government give presentation of BRONZE LORD SIVA STAUE 'S   to CERN laboratory ,to find our god particle's test.

PROCEDURE

one who wants to do this posture .mainly the person   with empty stomach ,and evacuate stools and urine .particularly free bowel movement is mainly presented when doing this posture .Small amount of water may be drink, ,take right place to perform this posture, without any disturbance ,.spread the bed sheet and yoga mate ,and stand with a focused mind with concentration ,take deep breath and exhale do this for at least three to five minutes.

Stand on the yoga mat with calm and focused mind.

Lift the left leg, and cross it right leg then the right leg slightly bend down.

Now left arm move to right wards of the body then the palm should be placed down to earth.

Then the right arm placed above the left arm wrist level, but, the palm of right arm should be focus to sky.

Maintain this posture up to one to two minute duration then come to normal stage.

Initial stage it difficult to perform this posture .but practical those who are practiced baratha natiyam dance, it is very easy.

Memory power and concentration will improved by this posture.

Stress and strain are relieved by this posture and this posture brings happy to the performer.

The leg and chest will get strength by this posture.

This one of the balance improved posture.

External genital organ get improved by this posture,

The yogig power will developed by this posture.

It improves the digestive power.

It reduced the abdominal fat and this posture is good for weight reduction.

CONTRAINDICATION

Those who are affected by sciatica ,cervical spondilities are advised to not perform this posture.

And elder with knee problem or other arthritic disorder not advice this posture,

1-Those who are suffered by hip and leg disorder or fracture.

2-During menstrual time.

3-Suffering from liver cirrhosis or stomach ulceration are not advised do this posture.

4-those who are pregnant.

5-any undergone abdominal surgery.

6- Bedridden.

7-after taking heavy meals and empty stomach.

8-before sleep this posture usually not advised.

9-person with any fracture in hand s and dislocation of the shoulder joint not advised to do this posture.

10-without proper sleep and diet you should not perform this posture.

11-befoer going to bed not advised to do this posture.

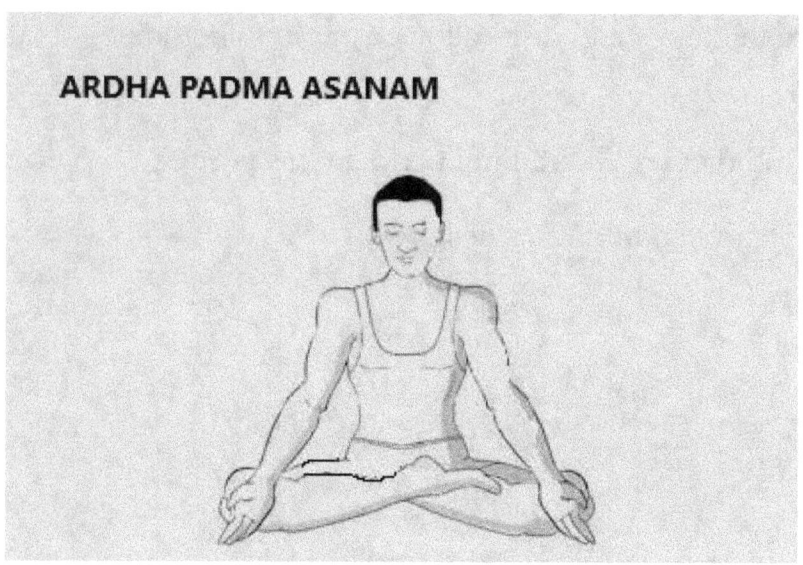

ARDHA PADMA ASANAM

DEFINATION

Dear reader today am going to illustrate about **ARDHA PADMASHANAM,** those who knows about **HINDHU** religion they must familiar with this posture because the most worship posture of god is seat on the lotus ,the great sages they perform majestic with this posture seated on a divine lotus,.

Latter in Buddhism and Jainism also the worship god seated on the lotus flower in this lotus posture,

The word meaning **ARDHA PADMASANAM** means joining of Three words one is **ARDHA** means ,half padma is lotus and asasanam means posture so it is called as half lotus posture.

one who wants to do this posture .mainly the person   with empty stomach ,and evacuate stools and urine .particularly free bowel movement is mainly presented when doing this posture .Small amount of water may be drink, ,take right place to perform this posture, without any disturbance ,.spread the bed sheet and yoga mate ,and stand with a focused mind with concentration ,take deep breath and exhale do this for at least three to five minutes.

And slowly sit on the mat with legs stretched out in front of you while keeping the spine erect position.

Slowly right knee bended and place it on the left thigh. The sole of the feet point upward and the heel is close to the groin region.

And keep it for three to five minute duration and come to normal posture .slowly

It one of the easiest posture to perform and this the variant type of padmasanam.

BENEFITS

It is very famous posture among the HINDHU sages and great saint many god form are in this posture only,

It will calms the mind .

Free from stress and strain.

 Improve the appetite .

Sub conscious mind is awakening concentration and memory power,

Restore our energy level.

It relieved the constipation and flatulence.

Provide strength to spine and waist region .

Pelvic muscle get strengthen.

Calve muscle hip muscle thigh muscles are get nourished and well developed.

Air holding capacity of lung got increased.

Relive from abdominal gas and flatulence .

Stimulate the live r by increasing the abdominal pressure it give good appetite also.

CONTRAINDICATION

And elder with knee problem or other arthritic disorder not advice this posture,.

1-Those who are suffered by hip and leg disorder or fracture.

2-During menstrual time.

3-Suffering from liver cirrhosis or stomach ulceration are not advised do this posture.

4-those who are pregnant.

5-any undergone abdominal surgery.

6- Bedridden.

7-after taking heavy meals and empty stomach.

8-before sleep this posture usually not advised.

9-person with any fracture in hand s and dislocation of the shoulder joint not advised to do this posture..

10-without proper sleep and diet you should not perform this posture .

11-befoer going to bed not advised to do this posture.

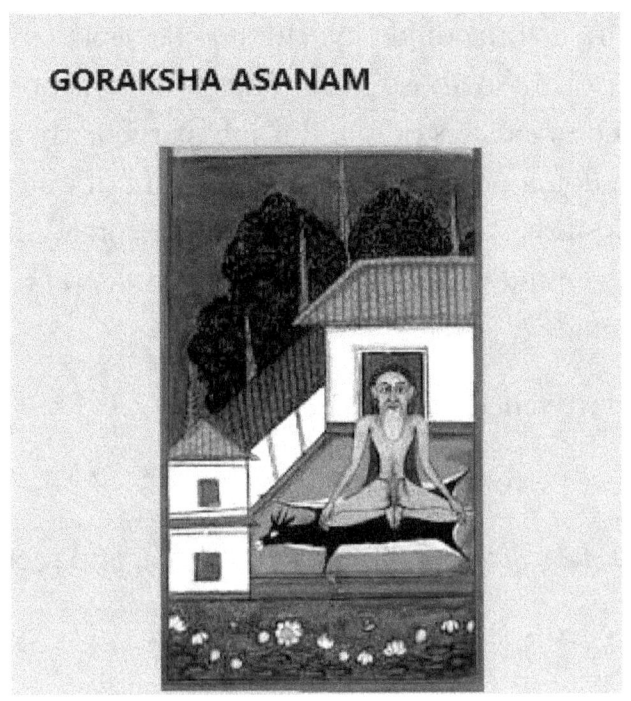

GORAKSHA ASANAM

Dear reader today am going to illustrate about *GORAKSHA ASANAM* the posture named as by great Hindu sage *GORAKANATHAR* who lived around 10century ,and he established the NATHA ancestry .the famous city GORAKPUR in India has put his name remembering .some authors are believed his tomb is situated near *NAGAPATTINAM DISTRICT in TAMILNADU* ,.there is one great tsunami attack in 2004 in east coastal area of Tamilnadu state ,but the tomb is not destroyed by the powerful waves of tsunami,.

The word meaning of goraksha is cowherd and asanam means posture .the cowherd posture is called as goraksha asanam .the great sage believed to sit in this posture only.

In early stage this posture is some difficulty. But regular practice and yogig person this posture very easy to perform. So ,those who wants to do this posture .mainly the person with empty stomach ,and evacuate stools and urine .particularly free bowel movement is mainly presented when doing this posture .Small amount of water may be drink, ,take right place to perform this posture, without any disturbance ,..spread the bed sheet and yoga mate ,and stand with a focused mind with concentration ,take deep breath and exhale do this for at least three to five minutes.

Sit on the yoga mat and stretched out the legs.

Take the right heel to near scrotal area .

The take the left heel to near left side of the scrotal area, and meet the two soul of the foot.

Then the two hand touched side of the knee joint area .

Now try to maintain two to three minute duration .and your familiar with pranayama you are advised to do it.

Then come to normal posture.

BENEFITS

This posture will help to awakening the **KUNDALINI** power from our body it is sited in **MOOLADHARAM.**

The lower limps are will get flexible .

The curvature of spinal cord will be corrected by this posture.

The external genital organ get strengthened, and it reduce the scrotal temperature will help to produce the sperm cell.

It reduces the flatus and constipation get relieved by this posture.

Stress and strain are removed by this posture.

Memory power will get improved by this posture.

Sub conscious mind is awakening concentration and memory power,

Restore our energy level.

Provide strength to spine and waist region.

Pelvic muscle get strengthen.

Calve muscle hip muscle thigh muscles are get nourished and well developed.

CONTRAINDICATION

And elder with knee problem or other arthritic disorder not advice this posture,

1-Those who are suffered by hip and leg disorder or fracture.

2-During menstrual time.

3-Suffering from liver cirrhosis or stomach ulceration are not advised do this posture.

4-those who are pregnant.

5-any undergone abdominal surgery.

6- Bedridden.

7-after taking heavy meals and empty stomach.

8-before sleep this posture usually not advised.

9-person with any fracture in hand s and dislocation of the shoulder joint not advised to do This posture.

10-without proper sleep and diet you should not perform this posture.

11-befoer going to bed not advised to do this posture.

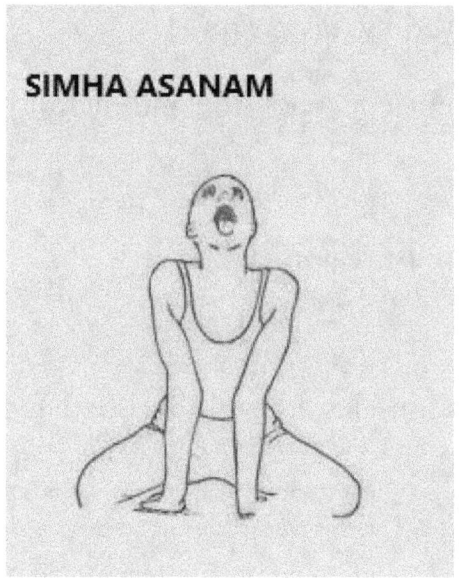

SIMHA ASANAM

DEFINATION

Dear reader today am going to illustrate about **SIMHA ASANAM** .the word meaning of simha means **lion** and asanam means posture ,so ,this posture is called as lion pose .it one of classical pose has mentioned in fourth and tenth century literature has describe about this posture ,among the other asanam this pose is mainly for MEDITATION purpose .one of eighteen century book **JOGA PRADIPIKA** has mentioned this pose as NARASIMHA ASANAM .because the word meaning **NARA** is human ,and asanam is simha asanam ,so it is called as **NARASIMHA ASANAM.**

one who wants to do this posture .mainly the person with empty stomach ,and evacuate stools and urine .particularly free bowel movement is mainly presented when doing this posture .Small amount of water may be drink, ,take right place to perform this posture, without any disturbance ,.spread the bed sheet and yoga mate ,and stand with a focused mind with concentration ,take deep breath and exhale do this for at least three to five minutes.

Stand on the yoga mat and slowly sit on knee bending posture

.Your buttocks are placed above the heels.

And stretched out the hand and touch the knee.

Then down your face look the earth, and extent your tongue out from mouth

. Normally the tongue tries to touch the chin.

And inhale the air large amount and exhale it.

BENEFITS

Tongue and throat muscle get strengthened by this posture.

This pose will help to reduce the body temperature.

Lung capacity has increased and reduces asthma and lung disorder.

Voice function gets improved by this pose, so singer try to this pose, will benefit to them.

It reduces the flatulence and constipation.

Provide strength to spine and waist region.

Pelvic muscle get strengthen.

Calve muscle hip muscle thigh muscles are get nourished and well developed.

Air holding capacity of lung got increased.

CONTRAINDICATION

Those who are affected by sciatica, cervical spondilities are advised to not perform this posture.

And elder with knee problem or other arthritic disorder not advice this posture,

1-Those who are suffered by hip and leg disorder or fracture.

2-During menstrual time.

3-Suffering from liver cirrhosis or stomach ulceration are not advised do this posture.

4-those who are pregnant.

5-any undergone abdominal surgery.

6- Bedridden.

7-after taking heavy meals and empty stomach.

8-before sleep this posture usually not advised.

9-person with any fracture in hand s and dislocation of the shoulder joint not advised to do this posture.

10-without proper sleep and diet you should not perform this posture .

11-before going to bed not advised to do this posture.

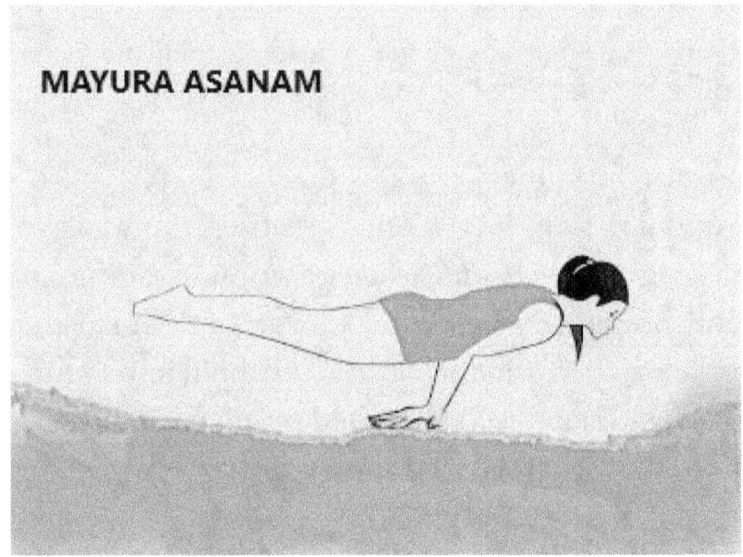

MAYURA ASANAM

DEFINATION

Dear reader today am going to illustrate about MAYURAASANAM ,it's joining of two letters the one is MAYURAM means the peacock and asanam means posture so the peacock posture is called as *MAYURA ASANAM* ,the peacock pose usually practice more than ten century .the *HATHA YOGA* PRADEEPIPKA one of the tenth century book has described this posture .and *VIMANA ARCHANA KALPA* is also described this posture .it is normally a non seated posture .it is sub divided in to some variants ,but, here it is not necessary to described here , only mayura asanam will described here .

It is non seated posture first time, when it is practiced it produced some strain to finger and arms .so initial precaution step to be taken. So those who wants to do this posture .mainly the person with empty stomach ,and evacuate stools and urine .particularly free bowel movement is mainly presented when doing this posture .Small amount of water may be drink, ,take right place to perform this posture, without any disturbance ,.spread the bed sheet and yoga mate ,and stand with a focused mind with concentration ,take deep breath and exhale do this for at least three to five minutes.

Lie in prone position on the yoga mat.

Then you have to mild breath, and place the palm on the earth near to side of the chest .

And lift the body by given pressure to the earth by the palm .

Maintain the straight position of the body,

And keep it for two to three minute duration .then come to normal posture.

Some of the sub variants are in this posture {pincha mayurasana, padma mayurasanam, syavanasana} are come under this type.

This posture is very helpful to reduce diabetic mellitus.

It stimulate the internal abdominal organ and induced the secretion,

.It provides good strength to arm and hips

It reduced the piles complaints.

It one of the energy relieving posture so, it will provide good digestion .

The abdominal muscle are tighten by this posture .

And reduced the abdominal fat .

This posture increases the lung capacity.

The vision power gets increased by this posture.

CONTRAINDICATION

Those who are affected by sciatica, cervical spondilities are advised to not perform this posture.

And elder with knee problem or other arthritic disorder not advice this posture,

1-Those who are suffered by hip and leg disorder or fracture.

2-During menstrual time.

3-Suffering from liver cirrhosis or stomach ulceration are not advised do this posture.

4-those who are pregnant.

5-any undergone abdominal surgery.

6- Bedridden.

7-after taking heavy meals and empty stomach.

8-before sleep this posture usually not advised .

9-person with any fracture in hand s and dislocation of the shoulder joint not advised to do this posture.

10-without proper sleep and diet you should not perform this posture.

11-befoer going to bed not advised to do this posture.

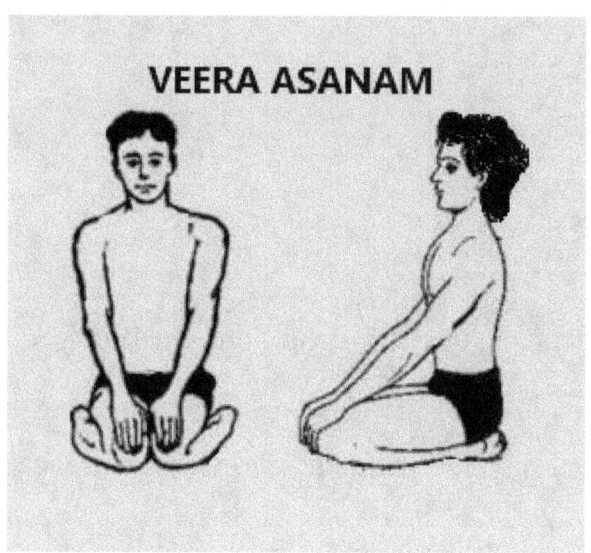

VEERA ASANAM

DEFINATION

Dear reader today am going to illustrate about **VIRA ASANAM** ,the word meaning of vira means warrior or hero is called as **VIRA** and ,asanam means posture ,so, the hero like posture is called as vira asanam ,its one of the ancient pose has mentioned in *Patanjalayogasastravivarana* (2.46-48) and the 13th century *Vasishthasamhita* .

so this posture is very familiar in ancient days .there is no chairs and table to sit in olden days ,if any function or meeting held a cotton mattress is proceeded, and the people sit in this posture on the mattress. So it is called as hero posture .now a days the chairs are produce laziness and disease to us but this asana is good for all people ,even if they sit for long duration.

PROCEDURE

one who wants to do this posture .mainly the person   with empty stomach ,and evacuate stools and urine .particularly free bowel movement is mainly presented when doing this posture .Small amount of water may be drink, ,take right place to perform this posture, without any disturbance ,.spread the bed sheet and yoga mate ,and stand with a focused mind with concentration ,take deep breath and exhale do this for at least three to five minutes. This one the sitting posture .so sit on the yoga mat in comfortable pose.

Then you to fold you left leg and the heel should be placed on the buttocks region .

Now the right leg fold the heel is placed under the buttocks .

The two souls are visible, and two knee are parallel position.

Keep it for ten to fifteen minute duration .then come to normal pose,

EYE exercise in this pose is very beneficial.

BENEFITS

It is very famous posture among the HINDHU sages and great saint many god forms are in this posture only,

It will calms the mind.

Free from stress and strain .

 Improve the appetite.

Sub conscious mind is awakening concentration and memory power,

Restore our energy level.

it relieved the constipation and flatulence.

CONTRAINDICATION

Those who are affected by sciatica ,cervical spondilities are advised to not perform this posture.

And elder with knee problem or other arthritic disorder not advice this posture,

1-Those who are suffered by hip and leg disorder or fracture.

2-During menstrual time.

3-Suffering from liver cirrhosis or stomach ulceration are not advised do this posture.

4-those who are pregnant.

5-any undergone abdominal surgery.

6- Bedridden.

7-after taking heavy meals and empty stomach.

8-before sleep this posture usually not advised.

9-person with any fracture in hand s and dislocation of the shoulder joint not advised to do this posture.

10-without proper sleep and diet you should not perform this posture.

11-befoer going to bed not advised to do this posture.

GARPA PIDA ASANAM

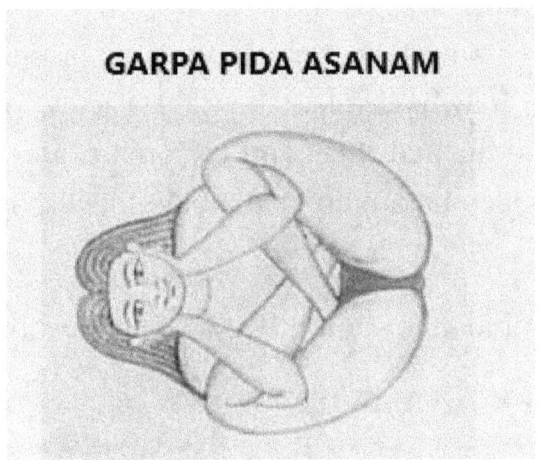

DEFINATION

Dear reader today am going to illustrate the GARBA PEEDA ASANAM is one of the famous asanam has mentioned in seventeenth century literature *BAHR-AL-HAYAT*, which was written by *GHAWATH*, and the nineteenth century book *SRITATTVANIDHI*, has illustrated about this pose .this posture is inverted variant of KURMAASSANAM .

The etymology of the word **GARBAPINDA ASANAM** is the word **GARBA** denote to uterus or womb and PINDA means foetus and ASANAM means posture .so, the posture resemble like sitting posture of the foetus in the mother womb is called as *GARBAPIPNDA ASANAM*.

It is one of the difficult pose to perform this posture but regular practice make it possible .so ,those who wants to do this posture .mainly the person with empty stomach ,and evacuate stools and urine .particularly free bowel movement is mainly presented when doing this posture .Small amount of water may be drink, ,take right place to perform this posture, without any disturbance ,.spread the bed sheet and yoga mate ,and stand with a focused mind with concentration ,take deep breath and exhale do this for at least three to five minutes.

And sit one yoga mat in calm mind take some **PRANAYAMA** {breathing exercise}.

Then you have to sit in **PADMASANA .POSE.**

Now you have entered your left hand to the folding left knee .

And like that right hand should be entered to right knee folding.

Slowly you have lie down on the yoga mat .then the two leg bring near to abdominal level and the arm should be touched the face.

Initially it is very difficult to perform, and keep it for one to two minute duration .then slowly release the hand, and come to normal posture.

BENEFITS

This pose stimulate the abdominal organs and regulate it function.

It strengthen the external genital organ .and improve the sperm production.

It relieve stress and strain, and reduce the mental tension.

Provide good sleep .

Body balance get improved by this posture .nervous system are work normal.

It provide good strength to arm and hips .

It reduced the piles complaints.

It one of the energy relieving posture so, it will provide good digestion.

The abdominal muscle are tighten by this posture .

And reduced the abdominal fat.

This posture increase the lung capacity.

CONTRAINDICATION

Those who are affected by sciatica ,cervical spondilities are advised to not perform this posture.

And elder with knee problem or other arthritic disorder not advice this posture,.

1-Those who are suffered by hip and leg disorder or fracture.

2-During menstrual time.

3-Suffering from liver cirrhosis or stomach ulceration are not advised do this posture.

4-those who are pregnant.

5-any undergone abdominal surgery.

6- Bedridden.

7-after taking heavy meals and empty stomach.

8-before sleep this posture usually not advised .

9-person with any fracture in hand s and dislocation of the shoulder joint not advised to do this posture.

10-without proper sleep and diet you should not perform this posture .

11-befoer going to bed not advised to do this posture,.

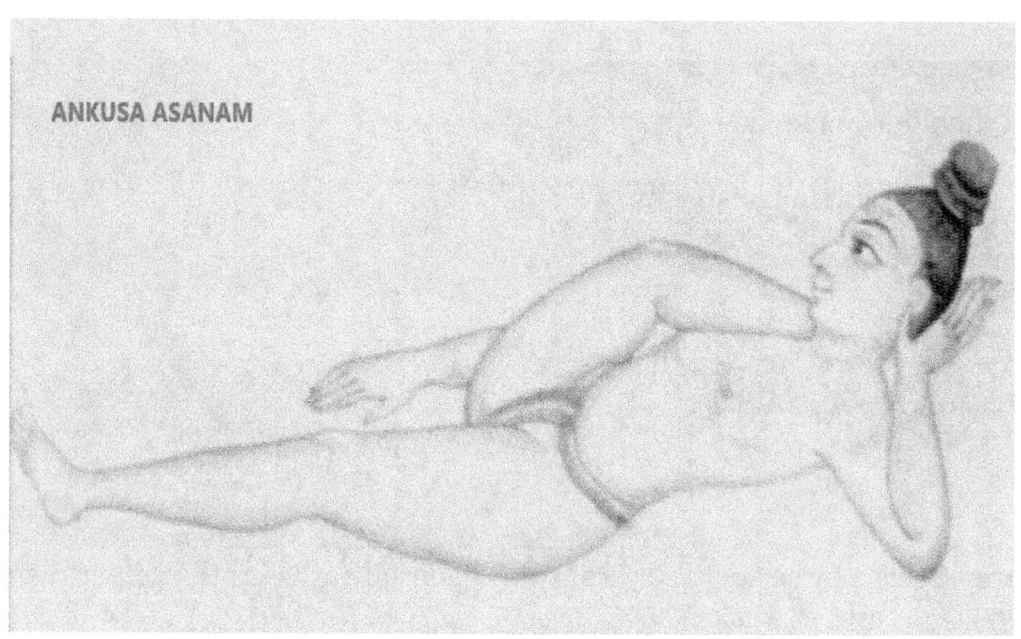

ANKUSA ASANAM

DEFINATION

Dear reader today am going to illustrate about BHAIRAVA ASANAM this pose otherwise called as *KAALABHAIRAVA ASANAM* .the LORD SIVA is present in this name in VARANASI, the kaala bhairava incarnation ,is one of the powerful incarnation taken by lord Siva, to destroyed the enemy and safe to sage and saint those who present or lived in VARANASI PLACE .the place is situated in north part of India on shore of GANGA RIVER .

The etymology of KAALA BHAIRAVA ASANAM is KAALA means blackness or time and BHAIRA means terrible, and ASANAM means posture .this posture was described in SRITHATHVANITHI one of eighteenth century book in the name of ANKUSA ASANAM, ANKURAM means the elephant goad an instrument to control the elephants and asanam means posture .

PROCEDURE

one who wants to do this posture .mainly the person with empty stomach ,and evacuate stools and urine .particularly free bowel movement is mainly presented when doing this posture .Small amount of water may be drink, ,take right place to perform this posture, without any disturbance ,.spread the bed sheet and yoga mate ,and stand with a focused mind with concentration ,take deep breath and exhale do this for at least three to five minutes.

Lie down on the yoga mat .and stretched out the legs.

Now you have lifted the right leg to above the level of head.

The right foot kept under the head like as pillow.

Then your left hand reached the right foot level behind the head .and join the left hand palm and right leg soul to meet, and formed like a prayer position.

The right arm kept on the earth parallel to the right leg.

Maintain this posture up to two three minute duration and come to normal stage.

BENEFITS

This one of the reclining pose is help to meditation for long time, but this is applicable only for yogig people only.

This pose provide strength to hip and waist region,

When give pressure on chest region by legs by changing the position the lung capacity and action may get increased by this posture.

The external genital organ get strengthen by this posture.

The PCOD problem in women reduced by this posture .and regulate the menstrual cycle.

Memory power and concentration get improved by this posture.

Provide good sleep.

Body balance get improved by this posture .nervous system are work normal.

It provides good strength to arm and hips.

It reduced the piles complaints.

It one of the energy relieving posture so, it will provide good digestion.

The abdominal muscle is tightening by this posture.

And reduced the abdominal fat.

CONTRAINDICATION

Those who are affected by sciatica, cervical spondilities are advised to not perform this posture.

And elder with knee problem or other arthritic disorder not advice this posture,

1-Those who are suffered by hip and leg disorder or fracture.

2-During menstrual time.

3-Suffering from liver cirrhosis or stomach ulceration are not advised do this posture.

4-those who are pregnant.

5-any undergone abdominal surgery.

6- Bedridden.

7-after taking heavy meals and empty stomach.

8-before sleep this posture usually not advised.

9-person with any fracture in hand s and dislocation of the shoulder joint not advised to do this posture.

10-without proper sleep and diet you should not perform this posture.

11-befoer going to bed not advised to do this posture.

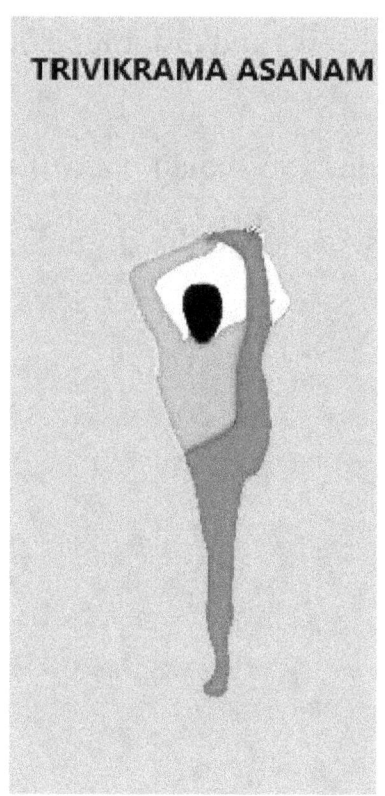

TRIVIKRAMA ASANAM

DEFINATION

Dear reader today am going to illustrate about *TRIVIKRAMAASANAM* ,now a days some authors named it as *dhuruvasana* .is named after famous sage *DHURUVASAR* ,he was familiar for his angriness ,he one of the raja rishi among the other sage that means king of all sages ,this posture was mentioned in *srithatthvanidhi* and *hathayogaabyasnithi* these are belongs to eighteenth century yoga literature .

The etymology of the word **TRIVIKRAMA ASANAM** is joining of three words one is **TRI** means three and **VIRAMA** means direction and asanam means posture, so the three directional postures is called as *trivikramasanam.*

PROCEDURE

One who wants to do this posture .mainly the person with empty stomach ,and evacuate stools and urine .particularly free bowel movement is mainly presented when doing this posture .Small amount of water may be drink, ,take right place to perform this posture, without any disturbance ,.spread the bed sheet and yoga mate ,and stand with a focused mind with concentration ,take deep breath and exhale do this for at least three to five minutes.

Stand erection posture on the yoga mat,

And slowly lift your left leg behind the back of the chest the knee is placed on near to the right shoulder or neck ,and the foot of the left leg to be focused parallel to the face direction .

Now you have to slightly bend the right knee.

Then you have to join your palm like prayer pose.

Keep this two to three minute duration then come to normal posture.

BENEFITS

This posture will help to awakening the **KUNDALINI** power.

The lower limp is will get flexible.

The external genital organ get strengthened, and it reduce the scrotal temperature will help to produce the sperm cell.

It reduce the flatus and constipation get relieved by this posture.

Stress and strain are removed by this posture.

Memory power will get improved by this posture.

Restore our energy level.

Provide strength to spine and waist region .

Pelvic muscle get strengthen .

Calve muscle hip muscle thigh muscles are get nourished and well developed.

Self balancing posture will improve by this posture.

CONTRAINDICATION

Those who are affected by sciatica ,cervical spondilities are advised to not perform this posture.

And elder with knee problem or other arthritic disorder not advice this posture,

1-Those who are suffered by hip and leg disorder or fracture.

2-During menstrual time.

3-Suffering from liver cirrhosis or stomach ulceration are not advised do this posture.

4-those who are pregnant.

5-any undergone abdominal surgery.

6- Bedridden.

7-after taking heavy meals and empty stomach.

8-before sleep this posture usually not advised .

9-person with any fracture in hand s and dislocation of the shoulder joint not advised to do this posture.

10-without proper sleep and diet you should not perform this posture .

11-befoer going to bed not advised to do this posture.

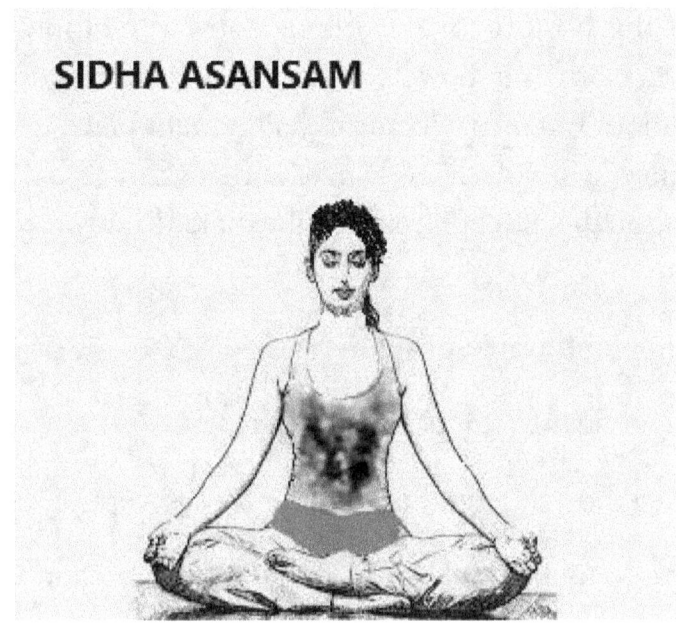

SIDHA ASANSAM

DEFINATION

Dear reader today am going to illustrate about SIDHA ASANAM is one of the oldest posture has mentioned in GORAKSHA SATAKA is one of oldest literature belong to ten century .some literature *HATHA YOGA PRADEEPIKA* is mentioned as *muktha asanam* .the etymology of the word sidha is perfect or obtain some super natural power that people is called as sidha ,and asanam means posture .sp the perfect pose to attain the yoga margam is called as *SIDDHA ASANAM or MUKTHA ASANAM .*

One of nineteenth century book *JOGA PRADEEPIKA* has illustrated this pose. in olden days this pose will performed on the tanned tiger skin .but in India hunting is banned .so dear reader kindly follow rules and regulation of your country ,strictly we have advised not to do.

one who wants to do this posture .mainly the person with empty stomach ,and evacuate stools and urine .particularly free bowel movement is mainly presented when doing this posture .Small amount of water may be drink, ,take right place to perform this posture, without any disturbance ,.spread the bed sheet and yoga mate ,and stand with a focused mind with concentration ,take deep breath and exhale do this for at least three to five minutes.

Sit on the yoga mat in comfortable position,

The right heel is placed near to the perennial area .

And the left leg is placed on the right leg and the foot is kept on the right thigh,

Then extent your arm to touch the border of the knee joint ,and maintain this pose for five to ten minute duration ,then come to normal position.

BENEFITS

It is very famous posture among the sages and great saint are in this posture only,

It will calms the mind.

Free from stress and strain .

 Improve the appetite .

Sub conscious mind is awakening concentration and memory power,

Restore our energy level.

it relieved the constipation and flatulence.

CONTRAINDICATION

And elder with knee problem or other arthritic disorder not advice this posture,

1-Those who are suffered by hip and leg disorder or fracture.

2-During menstrual time

3-Suffering from liver cirrhosis or stomach ulceration are not advised do this posture.

4-those who are pregnant.

5-any undergone abdominal surgery.

6- Bedridden.

7-after taking heavy meals and empty stomach.

8-before sleep this posture usually not advised .

9-person with any fracture in hand s and dislocation of the shoulder joint not advised to do this posture.

10-without proper sleep and diet you should not perform this posture.

11-befoer going to bed not advised to do this posture.

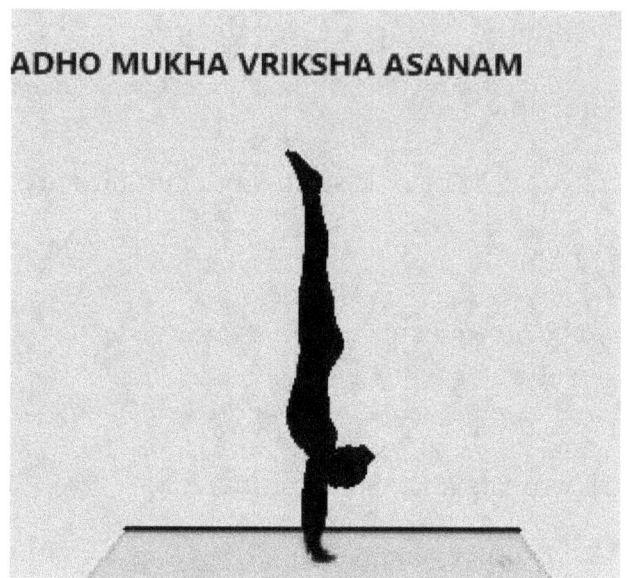

DEFINATION

Dear reader today am going to illustrate about ADHOMUKA VRIKSHA ASANAM ,is one of the posture has mentioned in the HATHA YOGA PRADEEPIKA one of the eighteen century literature has described this posture .

.The etymology ADHO MUKHA VRIKSHA ASANAM MEANS ,the word ADHO means downward direction MUKHA means posture ,and VRIKSHA mean TREE ,AND ASANAM means POSTURE ,so, the downward tree pose is called as ADHOMUKHA VRIKSHA ASANAM .this pose otherwise called as HAND STANDING pose .it is downward direction of the pose .

This pose very familiar in modern gymnastics and aerophics exercise, but it has mentioned and documented by the eighteenth century literature ,it is one of the downward pose .in initial stage it is very difficult ,but proper training give good result. So, those who wants to do this posture .mainly the person with empty stomach ,and evacuate stools and urine .particularly free bowel movement is mainly presented when doing this posture .Small amount of water may be drink, ,take right place to perform this posture, without any disturbance ,.spread the bed sheet and yoga mate ,and stand with a focused mind with concentration ,take deep breath and exhale do this for at least three to five minutes.

Stand on the yoga mat in a comfortable position.

Now you place the palm on the mat and try to lift the body in a vertical pose .it very difficult to perform ,first you have to select near to wall .then come to normal place.

Your hand is in rest position only, not bend the hand ,other wise your body weight lead to down on the earth'.

Keep it for two to three minute duration then come to normal position.

This posture is mainly balance our body.

Concentration and memory power will increased by this posture.

Vision power get improved by this posture.

It strength the arms .and flexibility get increased by this posture,

It relieved the flatulence and staged tools .and increase the appetite.

Heaviness in the abdomen and chest are reduced by this posture.

This pose one of the anti gravity pose so it improve the blood circulation to head and neck.

Those who are affected by sciatica, cervical spondilities are advised to not perform this posture.

And elder with knee problem or other arthritic disorder not advice this posture,

1-Those who are suffered by hip and leg disorder or fracture.

2-During menstrual time.

3-Suffering from liver cirrhosis or stomach ulceration are not advised do this posture.

4-those who are pregnant.

5-any undergone abdominal surgery.

6- Bedridden.

7-after taking heavy meals and empty stomach.

8-before sleep this posture usually not advised .

9-person with any fracture in hand s and dislocation of the shoulder joint not advised to do this posture.

10-without proper sleep and diet you should not perform this posture .

11-befoer going to bed not advised to do this posture.

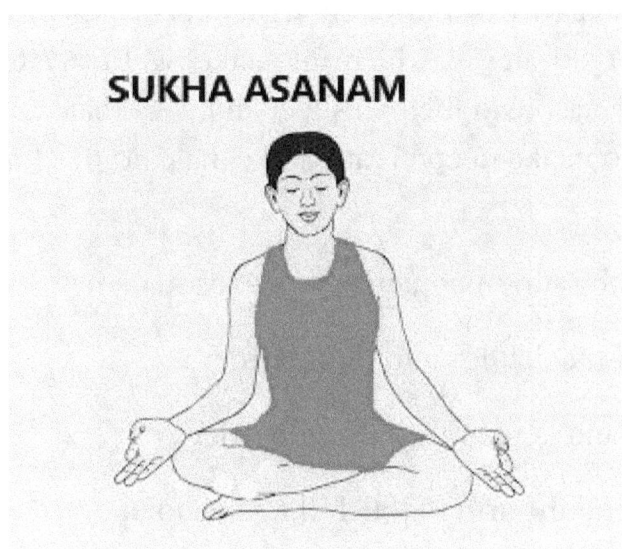

SUKHA ASANAM

DEFINATION

Dear reader today, am going to illustrate about SUKHA ASANAM is one the asanam is mentioned in the eighteenth century, literature SRITHATHVANIDHI and it has mentioned in the *DHARSANA UPANISAD* ,which was written in fourth century period particularly this pose indicate for meditation purpose ,.

The etymology of the word *SUKHASANAM* is the word meaning for SUKHA IS PLEASURE and asasnam is posture so it called as pleasure pose .

one who wants to do this posture .mainly the person   with empty stomach ,and evacuate stools and urine .particularly free bowel movement is mainly presented when doing this posture .Small amount of water may be drink, ,take right place to perform this posture, without any disturbance ,.spread the bed sheet and yoga mate ,and stand with a focused mind with concentration ,take deep breath and exhale do this for at least three to five minutes.

Sit on the yoga mat with calm mind ,and do pranayama.

Then you have to fold the left leg into right border .

And fold the right leg and kept in the left leg border .

Then you have to extend the arm to touch the knee joint .

Then keep it this pose for ten to fifteen minute duration ,in this time you have to perform meditation is ideal .

Then come to normal position.

BENEFITS

This pose mainly used for meditation purpose .

Memory power, and concentration will improved by this posture .

Those who are affected by anxiety, angry person this posture very useful to them.

This pose will balance between the mind and the body.

This pose one of the relaxing pose, so, after heavy work this pose regulate the muscle .

Sub conscious mind is awakening concentration and memory power,

Restore our energy level.

CONTRAINDICATION

Those who are affected by sciatica ,cervical spondilities are advised to not perform this posture.

And elder with knee problem or other arthritic disorder not advice this posture,

1-Those who are suffered by hip and leg disorder or fracture.

2-During menstrual time.

3-Suffering from liver cirrhosis or stomach ulceration are not advised do this posture.

4-those who are pregnant.

5-any undergone abdominal surgery.

6- Bedridden.

7-after taking heavy meals and empty stomach.

8-before sleep this posture usually not advised .

9-person with any fracture in hand s and dislocation of the shoulder joint not advised to do this posture.

10-without proper sleep and diet you should not perform this posture .

11-befoer going to bed not advised to do this posture.

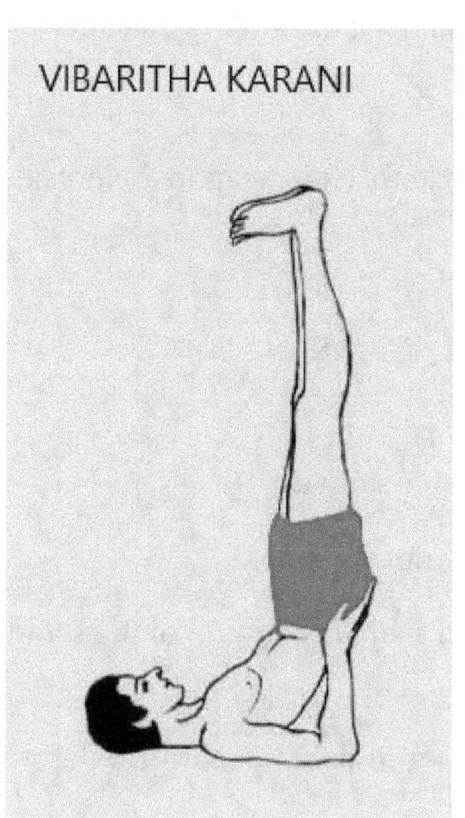

VIBARITHA KARANI

DEFINATION

Dear reader today am going to illustrate about *VIBARITHA KARANI ASANAM* ,is one of the oldest pose has practiced in long duration in India .in HATHA YOGA PRADEEPIKA has gives various name to this posture ,such as *NARAKASANAM ,KAPALASANAM*,etc but the eighteenth century book *JOGAPRADIPIKA* has demonstrated this pose very clearly .this pose very popular among the yogis because this pose will helpful to give the AMIRTHAM by the anti gravity force ,

The etymology of the word VIPARITHA KARANI is ,the word VIPARITHA means reverse or inverted and karani means activity .ASANAM means pose so the inverted pose is called as viparitha asanam .but here for which reason KARANI is the word added ,when perform this inverted pose we have to follow or do some PRANAYAMA THAT MEANS THE BREATHING EXCERCISE then only it will helpful to give the amirtham to the body .so this pose is called as VIPARITHA KARANI ASANAM.

PROCEDURE

This posture is same as sirasasanam so, initial stage is very difficult to do but regular practice it may helpful to do this pose. so ,one who wants to do this posture .mainly the person with empty stomach ,and evacuate stools and urine .particularly free bowel movement is mainly presented when doing this posture .Small amount of water may be drink, ,take right place to perform this posture, without any disturbance ,.spread the bed sheet and yoga mate ,and stand with a focused mind with concentration ,take deep breath and exhale do this for at least three to five minutes.

Lie down on the yoga mat on upward direction,

Then you have to lift your leg ,the hip is supported by hands ,the body is lifted as much as possible ,when do this posture along with PRANAYAMA it will raised the KUNDALI, then it reach the thousand petals lotus in brain and it secrete the NECTOR. or otherwise called as amirtham .it will supply to the body by anti gravitational force .this nectar will help full to yogi is give free from appetite and disease ,give youth and refreshment to the yogis .

And keep this pose for five to ten minute duration {those who are very familiar with yoga practice ,they only do this pose with breathing exercise ,so ,they only can able to perform this pose ten minute. duration}

Then slowly come to normal stage.

This pose very helpful those practice yoga with pranayama for awakening of KUNDALI ,this give some super natural power to yogis is called as ASTAMA SIDHI'S.

Regulate the blood flow.

Improve the digestion and appetite.

This one of the self balancing pose, the body is stand against the gravitational force .

The varicose veins are get cured by this pose.

This pose improve the testicular function, and cured the infertility.

This pose mainly used for meditation purpose .

Memory power, and concentration will improved by this posture .

Those who are affected by anxiety, angry person this posture very useful to them.

This pose will balance between the mind and the body .

Sub conscious mind is awakening concentration and memory power,

Restore our energy level.

CONTRAINDICATION

Those who are affected by sciatica ,cervical spondilities are advised to not perform this posture.

And elder with knee problem or other arthritic disorder not advice this posture,

1-Those who are suffered by hip and leg disorder or fracture.

2-During menstrual time.

3-Suffering from liver cirrhosis or stomach ulceration are not advised do this posture

4-those who are pregnant.

5-any undergone abdominal surgery.

6- Bedridden.

7-after taking heavy meals and empty stomach.

8-before sleep this posture usually not advised.

9-person with any fracture in hand s and dislocation of the shoulder joint not advised to do this posture.

10-without proper sleep and diet you should not perform this posture .

11-befoer going to bed not advised to do this posture.

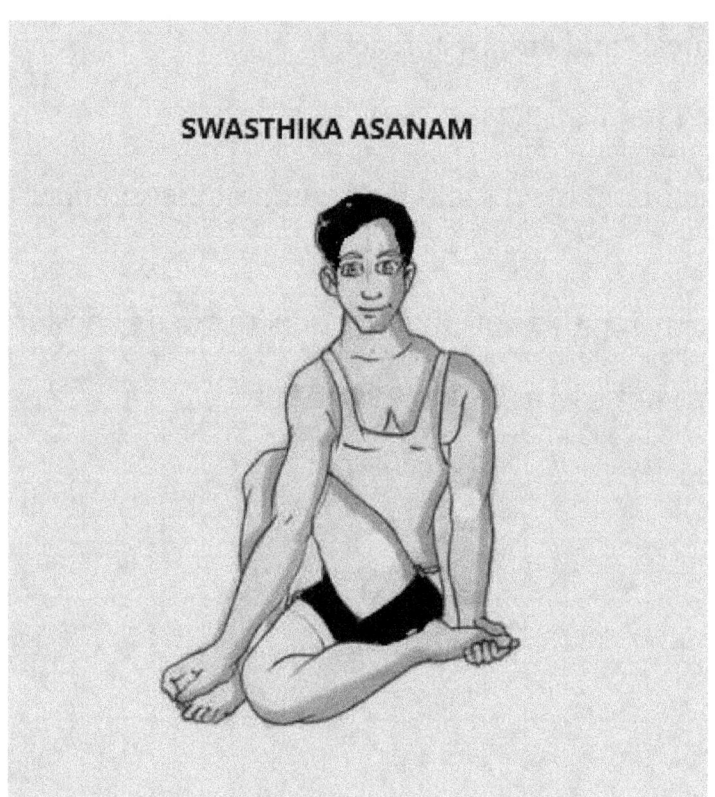

SWASTHIKA ASANAM

DEFINATION

Dear reader today am going to illustrate about the ***SWASTHIKA ASANAM*** ,the etymology of the word **swastika** means **auspicious** and asanam means posture ,so this posture is called as auspicious posture, some yogis do perform the meditation by this posture .this posture has illustrated in eighteenth century manual. And this pose also described in eighth century manual ***patanjalayogasastravivarana*** and in the tenth century vimanarcanakalpa.also mentioned this pose .

This posture is very easy to perform .but, basic premonitory method is very essential for all posture .those who wants to do this posture .mainly the person with empty stomach ,and evacuate stools and urine .particularly free bowel movement is mainly presented when doing this posture .Small amount of water may be drink, ,take right place to perform this posture, without any disturbance ,.spread the bed sheet and yoga mate ,and stand with a focused mind with concentration ,take deep breath and exhale do this for at least three to five minutes.

Sit on the yoga mat in a comfortable pose.

Then you have to extend your leg, then fold the right leg and kept under the left leg,

Now you have to fold the left leg and the foot is backwards to nearby the buttocks.

Now you have to extend the arm, the right arm kept on the right knee.

And left arm kept on the right leg ankles, and maintain this pose for two to three minute ,

And slowly come to normal stage.

BENEFITS

This pose is very helpful for doing the meditation.

Memory power, and concentration will improved by this posture .

Those who are affected by anxiety, angry person this posture very useful to them.

This pose will balance between the mind and the body.

Sub conscious mind is awakening concentration and memory power,.

Restore our energy level.

, This pose provide strength to hip and waist region,

When give pressure on chest region by legs by changing the position the lung capacity and action may get increased by this posture.

The external genital organ get strengthen by this posture.

The PCOD problem in women reduced by this posture .and regulate the menstrual cycle.

CONTRAINDICATION

Those who are affected by sciatica, cervical spondilities are advised to not perform this posture.

And elder with knee problem or other arthritic disorder not advice this posture,

1-Those who are suffered by hip and leg disorder or fracture

.2-During menstrual time.

3-Suffering from liver cirrhosis or stomach ulceration are not advised do this posture.

4-those who are pregnant.

5-any undergone abdominal surgery.

6- Bedridden.

7-after taking heavy meals and empty stomach.

8-before sleep this posture usually not advised.

9-person with any fracture in hand s and dislocation of the shoulder joint not advised to do this posture.

10-without proper sleep and diet you should not perform this posture.

11-befoer going to bed not advised to do this posture.

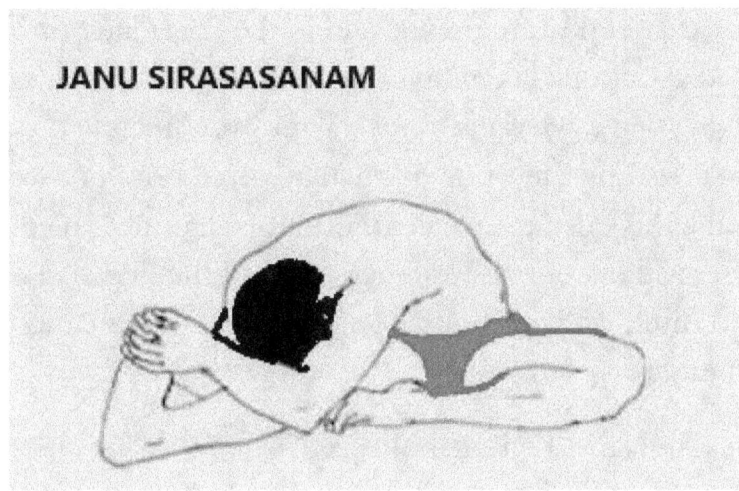

JANU SIRASASANAM

DEFINATION

Dear reader today am going to illustrate about *JANU SIRAS ASANAM* .THE WORD MEANING FOR JANU is knee and SIRAS means head and the last word is asanam this means posture, so it called as JANUSIRASASANAM when the head is take rest on the knee is called as JANUSIRASSASANAM .dear reader there is two knee but only one head is there, so preferably place the head on the top of left knee joint is indicated.

This one of the very easiest posture mentioned in the yogig literature but thre is some premonitory method should be taken before going to practiser any posture is essential and very important one ,so one who wants to do this posture .mainly the person , with empty stomach ,and evacuate stools and urine .particularly free bowel movement is mainly presented when doing this posture .Small amount of water may be drink, ,take right place to perform this posture, without any disturbance ,.spread the bed sheet and yoga mate ,and stand with a focused mind with concentration ,take deep breath and exhale do this for at least three to five minutes.

Slowly sit on the mat and stretched the both legs..

Then the soul of the right leg has to be placed near to the inguinal areas

.And try to hold the left feet by palm of the two hand in a interlock position,

Then bend forwardly and rest the head on the top of the left knee.

Keep it up for two to three minutes, and then come to normal position.

BENEFITS

It reduces the fat in our body particularly abdominal fat get reduced by this posture.

Internal organ are get benefitted by this posture.

The spleen and kidney's are do their normal functions.

This posture reduces the flatulence and constipation.

It is one of the energetic posture it provide whole day refreshment.

The sexual power will also get improved by this posture.

CONTRAINDICATION

Those who are affected by lumbar bone disorder are advised to not perform this posture.

And elder with knee problem or other arthritic disorder not advice this posture,

1-Those who are suffered by hip and leg disorder or fracture.

2-During menstrual time.

3-Suffering from liver cirrhosis or stomach ulceration are not advised do this posture.

4-those who are pregnant.

5-any undergone abdominal surgery.

6- Bedridden.

7-after taking heavy meals and empty stomach.

8-before sleep this posture usually not advised .

9-person with any fracture in hand s and dislocation of the shoulder joint not advised to do this posture.

10-without proper sleep and diet you should not perform this posture .

11-befoer going to bed not advised to do this posture.

12-urinary bladder stone are not advised to do this posture.

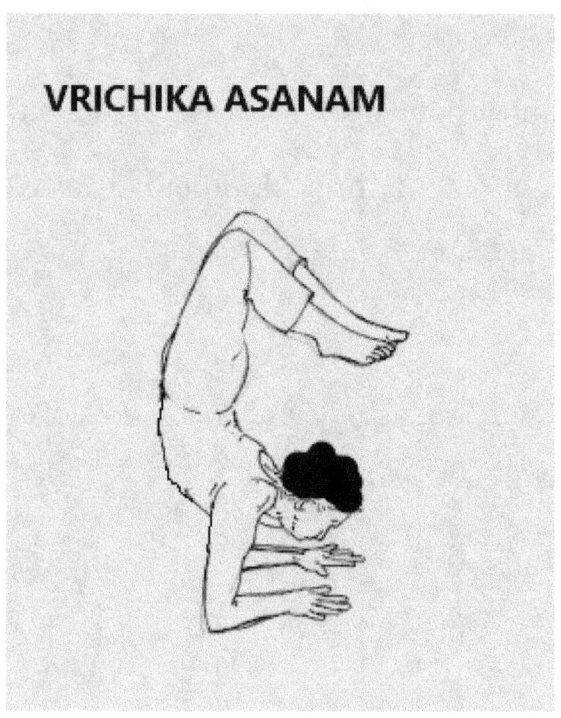

VRICHIKA ASANAM

Dear reader today am going to illustrate about **_VRICHIKAASANAM,_** it is a combination of two word's one is **vrichika this** meaning is indicate the scorpion. In normally a person should stand like scorpion position. ASANAM means posture, so it called as deep stretched standing like scorpion position is called as VRICHIKASANAM.

one who wants to do this posture .mainly the person   with empty stomach ,and evacuate stools and urine .particularly free bowel movement is mainly presented when doing this posture .Small amount of water may be drink, ,take right place to perform this posture, without any disturbance ,.spread the bed sheet and yoga mate ,and stand with a focused mind with concentration ,take deep breath and exhale do this for at least three to five minutes.

Then sit on the yoga mat on knee down position, placed the heel in near to the perineum areas .

And put the hand in front of the knee and lift the whole body the leg in upward direction and erectly.

Then slowly bend the hip and bend the knee downward direction and the foot touches the head region and keep it for thirty second duration.

And come to normal position.

Then sit calmly for two minutes .the reader not advised to stand immediately because more blood is flow to head r area. When you will stand some giddiness will occur, so the reader is precaution for this posture .

BENEFITS

The arm and forearm get strengthened by this posture .

Flexibility and balance of the body will get improved by this posture,

Reduced the haemorrhoids and constipation etc.

Improve the blood circulation to the limps.

The hip is get strengthened and internal organs are get benefitted by this posture.

Brain activity gets improved and it boosts the memory and concentration.

The stress and strain are get relieved by this posture.

When doing this posture in early morning, it gives refreshment to the whole day.

CONTRAINDICATION

Those who are affected by sciatica ,cervical spondilities are advised to not perform this posture.

And elder with knee problem or other arthritic disorder not advice this posture,

Those who are affected by neurological disorder.

Affected by vertigo giddiness etc not advised to do this posture,.

1-Those who are suffered by hip and leg disorder or fracture.

2-During menstrual time.

3-Suffering from liver cirrhosis or stomach ulceration are not advised do this posture.

4-those who are pregnant.

5-any undergone abdominal surgery.

6- Bedridden.

7-after taking heavy meals and empty stomach.

8-before sleep this posture usually not advised .

9-person with any fracture in hand s and dislocation of the shoulder joint not advised to do this posture.

10-without proper sleep and diet you should not perform this posture .

11-before going to bed not advised to do this posture.

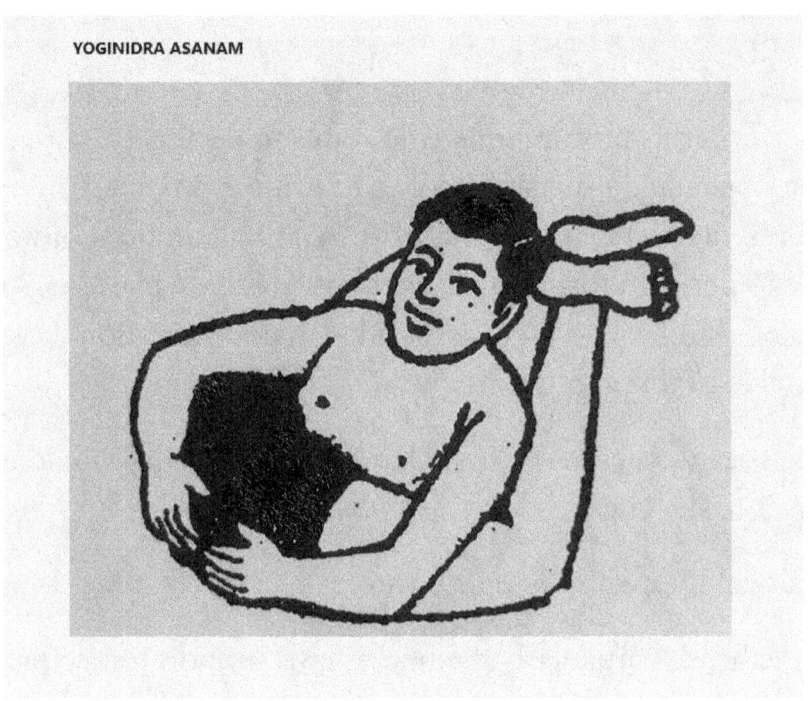

YOGINIDRA ASANAM

DEFINATION

Dear reader today am going to illustrate about YOGI NIDRA ASANAM, it is a combination of three word one is YOGI this meaning is indicate that, who is in the master of the yoga science and well versed in all type of posture and ready to attain moksham prapthi is called as yogi and the word *NIDRA* means Sleep ASANAM means posture ,so it called as the sleep of a yogig person is called as *YOGINIDRAASANAM.* This posture is found on the stone sculpture of the classical Hindu temples. When place the head in between the two legs so in modern days somebody is called *DVI PADA SIRASASANAM.* The pose is illustrated in an 18th century painting of the 8 yoga chakras in Mysore palace paintings.

This posture is very helpful to awakening the power of the KUNDLAINI power from the mooladharam. Even though it is very difficult to perform this posture but it provide many benefit s to our body and the mind.

PROCEDURE

It is very difficult to perform this posture .one who wants to do this posture .mainly the person with empty stomach ,and evacuate stools and urine .particularly free bowel movement is mainly presented when doing this posture .Small amount of water may be drink, ,take right place to perform this posture, without any disturbance ,.spread the bed sheet and yoga mate ,and stand with a focused mind with concentration ,take deep breath and exhale do this for at least three to five minutes.

Slowly lie down on the yoga mat, come into the Savaasanas after that breathe in along with keeping your right knees to the chest.

 then the person lift the right leg with the right hand

Placed the leg under the head, particularly the heel is give support to occipital region of the head .

Then you have to lift the left leg and bending, placed under the right leg .now the head is placed exactly in between the two heels,

{previously I tell that the head is placed on the right leg. now I tell that the head is placed in between two heels ,you placed the head in right heels otherwise the head will go down, your unable to lift the head when you bend right leg ,}

Then you have locked the palm in near to the buttocks region.

Then keep it for one to two minutes, then slowly relieved from the posture and come to normal stage.

This posture will helpful to awakening the power of KUNDALI.

The stress and strain are relieved.

Memory power will improved by this posture.

Some authors put some mudra for this posture to prevent the escape of the prana but perform one to two minute duration, it is not necessary for us only yogig person will do this posture for long time so they put *mudra* for this posture.

External genital organs are get strengthened, the sexual power will also get improved by this posture

Lung capacity is increased by this posture.

CONTRAINDICATION

Those who are affected by sciatica, cervical spondilities are advised to not perform this posture.

And elder with knee problem or other arthritic disorder not advice this posture,

1-Those who are suffered by hip and leg disorder or fracture.

2-During menstrual time.

3-Suffering from liver cirrhosis or stomach ulceration are not advised do this posture.

4-those who are pregnant.

5-any undergone abdominal surgery.

6- Bedridden.

7-after taking heavy meals and empty stomach.

8-before sleep this posture usually not advised .

9-person with any fracture in hand s and dislocation of the shoulder joint not advised to do this posture.

10-without proper sleep and diet you should not perform this posture .

11-Befoer going to bed not advised to do this posture.

12-Those who are having hypertension and cardiovascular problem not advised to perform this posture.

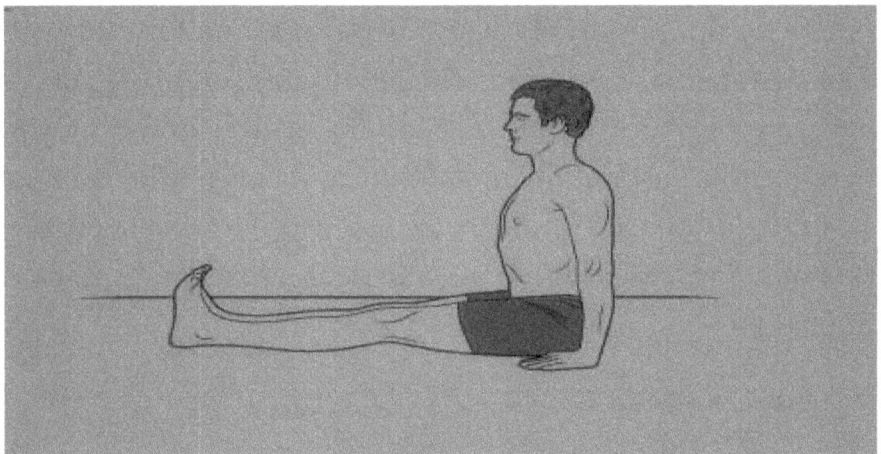

DEFINATION

The 19 'the century text ***SRITATVANIDHI*** has described this posture ,but in classical books like *hatha yoga pradipika* are not described about this posture ,so, Dear reader now am going to described about the danda asanam ,in Sanskrit language the word meaning ***DANDA*** is stick or staff and asanam means posture ,the stick like posture is called as dandaasanam .so authors are included this posture in to ***SURYA NAMASKAR*** posture ,but others are give opinion that it is different one .

It is not very difficult one to do this posture it is very easy to perform this one ,but the precaution is same for all posture, so those who wants to do this posture .mainly the person with empty stomach ,and evacuate stools and urine .particularly free bowel movement is mainly presented when doing this posture .Small amount of water may be drink, ,take right place to perform this posture, without any disturbance ,.spread the bed sheet and yoga mate ,and stand with a focused mind with concentration ,take deep breath and exhale do this for at least three to five minutes.

Slowly sit on the mat in a erect posture .

Stretch out the leg make sure that the two foots are parallel to each other and give mild pressure on the earth by the buttocks and face the head in upward position looks the roof of the building.

Keep erect the spine without curving the body .sit on erect position.

Keep it for two to three minute duration.

Then slowly come to normal position.

BENEFITS

This posture provides strength to chest muscle.

The holding capacity of air in lungs gets increased.

The children's those who are affected by asthma they quickly get relief from this posture.

The abdominal wall gets tightened, so, this asana prevent the herniation disorder.

The stress and strain are getting relieved by this posture.

When doing this posture in early morning, it gives refreshment to the whole day.

Legs, thighs, ankles, and heels are actively engaged in the practice of this posture so the patient who are affected by sciatica disorder arc gct sonly relieved by this posture.

It improves the digestive activity.

CONTRAINDICATION

1-Those who are suffered by hip and leg disorder or fracture.

2-During menstrual time.

3-Suffering from liver cirrhosis or stomach ulceration are not advised do this posture.

4-those who are pregnant.

5-any undergone abdominal surgery.

6- Bedridden.

7-after taking heavy meals and empty stomach.

8-before sleep this posture usually not advised .

9-person with any fracture in hand s and dislocation of the shoulder joint not advised to do this posture.

10-without proper sleep and diet you should not perform this posture .

11-befoer going to bed not advised to do this posture.

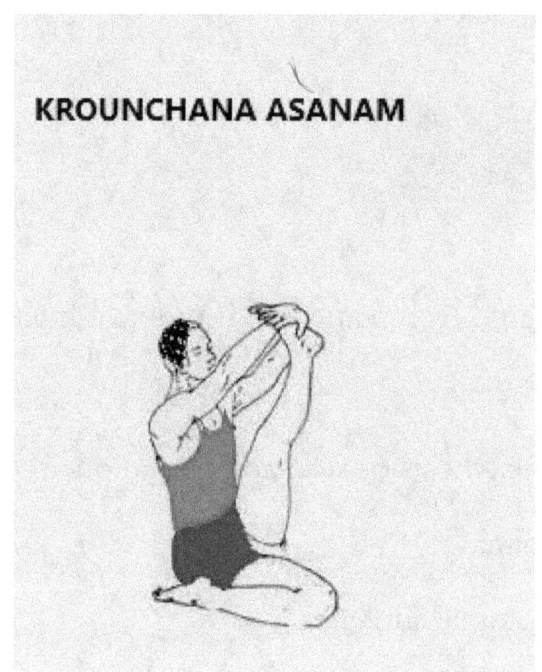

KROUNCHANA ASANAM

DEFINATION

Dear reader today am going to illustrate about **KROUNCHANA ASANAM** ,the etymology of the word **KROUNCHANA** means *heron* and the word asanam means posture .this pose was described in nineteenth century literature *JOGA PRADIPIKA* .and this pose was described in HATHA RATNAVALLI is one of the seventeenth century literature ,in this manual only eighty four kind of posture has mentioned .

PROCEDURE

This one of very easiest posture to perform in sitting position. so, those who wants to do this posture .mainly the person with empty stomach ,and evacuate stools and urine .particularly free bowel movement is mainly presented when doing this posture .Small amount of water may be drink, ,take right place to perform this posture, without any disturbance ,.spread the bed sheet and yoga mate ,and stand with a focused mind with concentration ,take deep breath and exhale do this for at least three to five minutes.

Sit on the yoga mat and stretched out your leg, and sit like ' L 'shaped .

Then you have to fold your left leg and the heel is kept near to the buttocks, the foot is facing upward direction.

Now you have to lift the right leg, and try to catch foot by two palms,

Then you have rest your leg on the right thigh,

Maintain this pose for two to three minute duration then come to normal position.

BENEFITS

This pose is very helpful for women those who suffering by uterine disorder and regulate the menstrual cycle.

It gives strength to external genital organ.

This pose tightens the abdominal muscle.

It reduces the fat in our body particularly abdominal fat get reduced by this posture.

Internal organ are get benefitted by this posture.

The spleen and kidney's are do their normal function.

This posture reduces the flatulence and constipation.

It is one of the energetic posture it provide whole day refreshment.

The sexual power will also get improved by this posture.

CONTRAINDICATION

Those who are affected by sciatica, cervical spondilities are advised to not perform this posture.

And elder with knee problem or other arthritic disorder not advice this posture,.

1-Those who are suffered by hip and leg disorder or fracture.

2-During menstrual time.

3-Suffering from liver cirrhosis or stomach ulceration are not advised do this posture.

4-those who are pregnant.

5-any undergone abdominal surgery.

6- Bedridden.

7-after taking heavy meals and empty stomach.

8-before sleep this posture usually not advised.

9-person with any fracture in hand s and dislocation of the shoulder joint not advised to do this posture.

10-without proper sleep and diet you should not perform this posture .

11-befoer going to bed not advised to do this posture.

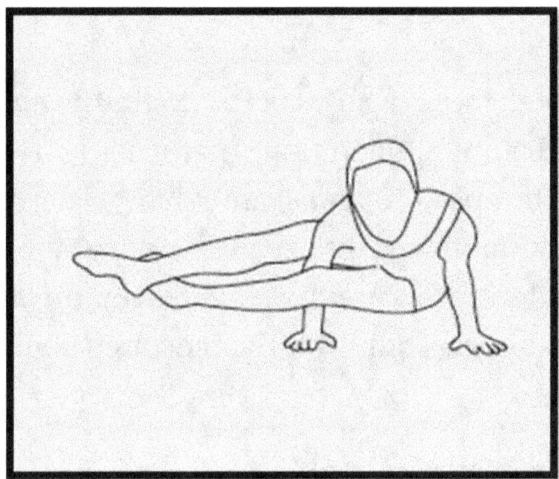

DEFINATION

Dear reader today am going to illustrate about ASTAVAKRAASANAM ,it is a combination of two word one is ASTA this meaning is in Sanskrit language EIGHT, and VAKKRAM means bend or curvature ASANAM means posture ,so it called as eight bending posture or eight curvature posture ,it is very difficulty one at initial stage, we have to advised not perform this posture ,but this posture is very famous in yogig culture, many authors are indicate this posture benefits ,in modern form of gymnastics this posture is performed now a days.

This posture is very difficult one ,those who wants to do this posture .mainly the person with empty stomach ,and evacuate stools and urine .particularly free bowel movement is mainly presented when doing this posture .Small amount of water may be drink, ,take right place to perform this posture, without any disturbance ,.spread the bed sheet and yoga mate ,and stand with a focused mind with concentration ,take deep breath and exhale do this for at least three to five minutes. this procedure is for all posture should be taken as pre operatory preparation.

First you have to sit on the yoga mat comfortably .

And put right arm in between two legs, then locked your legs by keeping the hand in between two legs.

Place your two palms on the earth in equal line.

And lift the body by hand during this lift the locked leg should be in the right hand.

During this posture the hip and should be in 'L' shaped.

Keep this posture up to one to two minute duration.

BENEFITS

It is one of the good posture to reduce the fat on our body .

Stamina get improved.

Spinal cord and spinal supporting muscle get benefitted by this posture.

Major internal organs are present in the right side of the abdomen like liver kidney ,lungs pancreases head ,female urinary bladder etc are got benefitted by this posture,

It increase the production of gastric juice and bile juice our appetites will increases and the digestion capacity will increase.

Tones the abdominal walls and thighs .

CONTRAINDICATION

Without proper training perform this posture will create some problem so. dear reader ,we have to advice please take proper precaution method,

Those who are affected by head and neck disorder are advised to not perform this posture.

And elder with knee problem or other arthritic disorder not advice this posture,

1-Those who are suffered by hip and leg disorder or fracture.

2-During menstrual time.

3-Suffering from liver cirrhosis or stomach ulceration are not advised do this posture.

4-those who are pregnant.

5-any undergone abdominal surgery.

 6- Bedridden.

7-after taking heavy meals and empty stomach.

8-person with any fracture in hand s and dislocation of the shoulder joint not advised to do this posture.

9-without proper sleep and diet you should not perform this posture .

10-person with hyper tension or cardio vascular problem not advised to do this posture.

PATHANJALLI YOGA SUTRAM

Among ancient literature about the science of yoga THE PATHANJALI YOGA SUTRAM is authentically one ,It was believed to written in 400ce there are 196 verses are described the total science of the yoga ,it is divided in to four major chapter named as follow,

1-SAMADHI PADHAM

2-SADHANA PADHAM

3-VIBUTI PADAM

4-KAIVALYA PADAM

SAMADHI PADHAM

Is first chapter in pathanjali yoga sutram text it contain 51 verses, this first chapter described about the primary preparation for yoga practices ,mainly it deals about concentration method ,with out proper concentrate sage deal in this chapter about the concentration .The other authors are explain this chapter as concentration ,when going to perform any work like study,playing,working ,cooking driving etc all work need concentration ,whenever doing any work main concentration is needed ,but the yoga is the main work to be given to mind so the meaning concentration is not suitable for this chapter.

In my view the word meaning SAMADHI is provide name peace or calm nature to mind ,when sitting without any works we can't concentrate anything when our mouth is closed our mind will speak ,and ruminate about past thinking ,and brief imagination about our future life ,it may sweet able or threat able it depend upon the individual.

That type of peaceful or calm full preparation is needed for practising the YOGA.thats way the great sage PATHANJALI put name as SAMADHI I for his first chapter ,*padam* means portion or lesson .so it provide meaning of calm or peaceful .

This chapter is a pre-operative for practising the yoga, in this area he described about mind and its nature ,types of knowledge ,knowledge perception method .how the impurity occur to the mind or add to the mind ,how desire will create the impurity to the mind also explain in this chapter .

How to concentrate our mind with PRANAVA MANDHIRAM, and usage also mentioned in this chapter obstacles for attain the peacefulness and its solution ,stabilizing the mind, and maintain a clear sound full way of mind also explained in this chapter.

SADHANA PADHAM

In this chapter he deals about practice of yoga .it contain 55 sutras ,it is broadly divided in to two types KRIYA YOGA and other one is ASTANGA YOGA .

IN KRIYA YOGA he deals about to attain the salvation by, NIYAMA ,TABAS,and ISHVARA PRANIDHANAM ,etc.

In astanga yoga he deals about eight fold of yoga YAMA ,NIYAMA ,ASANA,PRANAYANAM ,PRATHYAHARAM ,DHARANAI,DHYANAM,SAMADHI.

VIBUTI PADAM

The word meaning of VIBUTHI PADHAM means POWER or SIDDHIS attained by the hard work of the eight fold of the yoga, the person can attained the power some super natural effect .there are 56 verses are described here.

KAIVALYA PADAM

In this chapter there are 36 verse described here ,the etymology of the word KAIVALYA means ISOLOTION or SEPERATION of a person different from other activity to attain salvation purpose .

After the period of pathanjali ,one of the notable text is HATHA YOGA PRADHEEPIKA ,the etymology of the word HA means it denote to sun ,and the word THA represent MOON and PRADEEPIKA means brightness .There is two NADI called as IDA and PINGALA is travelled in crisscross section and reach to kapalam [brain] ,this two NADI always travel like serpent and it start from MOOLADHARAM ,dear reader you will also check this NADI's function by a simple test ,take your index finger very close to two nostrils and slowly exhale the breath ,the air will comes out from one nostrils in force the other in mild ,after thirty minute duration the air will comes out forcefully in other opening .this cycle running throughout our life .During the two nadis travel in crisscross method they met six point is called ADHARAM ,this run as a physiological cycle ,the yogi only stop this nadi in brain or thousand pedals lotus ,in this time a brighter light comes out ,and flow the nectar ,to inner part of the tongue .this great explanation are hidden in behind the title HATHA YOGA PRADEEPIKA ,this book was written in 15th century ad by swamy swatmarma .

This manual have four chapters.

The first chapter described about the POSTURE,

Chapter Two he deal with SAD KARMA and BREATHING EXERCISE .

Chapter 3RD he deals about some SYMPOLS and BONDAGE , and in

Chapter Four: he described about CONCENTRATION.

GHERANDA SAMHITHA

Although there are only 32 postures in "Gheranda Samhita," Gheranda explains that there are as many asana as there are species on the planet, every animal pose consider as a ASANAM [posture] but there are eighty four basic posture is there . It is stated that it is essential to include at least one inversion in every daily practice of yoga.

The GHERANDA SAMHITHA text basically start as a conversation between master GHERANDA and his student CHANDA .

The student asked about various question regarding about the posture the master described briefly .it may be written in seventeenth century ad .The area may be present in northeast part of the India. the GHERANDA SAMHITHA have seven chapter with 351 verses .

The master GHERANDA give very detailed about the yoga science and step by step he narrate to his student CHANDA .

SAD KARMA

Meaning of sad karma is six essential procedures to purpose of cleaning our body, without body purification the postural exercise can create some problem, so body cleaning is essential.

ASANAM- Meaning comfortable sitting.

MUDRA- Showing some symbols during asanam performance.

PRATHYAHARAM Means controlling the mind .

PRANAYAMA- Means breathing exercise .

DHYANAM- Means meditation .

SAMADHI - Means TOMP to attain salvation purpose .

GORAKSH SAMHITHA

The sage GORAKAR has believed to he is the establisher of the NATH PARAMBARAI,he may lived in eleventh century ad .but some study shows that, he is apart from the human origin ,he take rebirth in periodical .he his disciples named as MATSYENDRA NATH .he may lived in GARBAGIRI ,

IN TAMIL sidha system of medicine he wrote some sidha text.

His Samadhi [TOMB] is situated in GORAKPUR.

He is in the master of the yoga science, and Indian medicine, the GORAKSHA SAMHITHA has elaborately described about the yoga science.

ANNEXURE

ASANAS	-POSTURE
DHYANAM	-MEDITATION
SARPAM	-COPRA
TRIKONAM	-TRI ANGLE
KONA	-ANGLE
SURYA	-SUN
VEDHA	-ANCIENT SCIENCE
UTKATA	-FURIUOS
KAN	-EYE
NAMASKARAM	-WORSHIP
SANEESWARAR	-REPRESENT SATURN PLANET
PARAMPARAI	- FAMILY TRATITION
SAMADHI	-TOMP
SIDHA NATURAL POWER LIVING IN	- PERSON WITH SUPER
	TAMILNADU .
MATSHYA SUCH AS CROCODILE, FISH ETC	-WATER LIVING BEINGS
DHYANAM	-MEDITATION
PRANAYAMA	- BREATHING EXCERCISE

MUDRA	- Showing some symbols during asanam performance.
PRATHYAHARAM	- controlling the mind .
KARMA	- ACTION OR FUNCTION
SAD	-SIX
KAIVALYA	- ISOLOTION
VIBUTHI	- POWER
SUTRAM/SULOGAM	-VERSES ,POEM.
ASTAM	- EIGHT
VAKRAM	- BEND
DANDA	- STICK
YOGI	- MASTER IN YOGA SCIENCE
KUNDALI	- POWER WHICH WAS SLEEP IN PERENIUM REGION
VAJRAM	-DIAMOND
SAVA	-CORPSE
MAKARAM	- CAPRICORN-CROCODILE
PAVANUM	- WIND
KOSTA	-STOMACH
SAKA	- LIMP
BALA	- CHILD
SARVANGA	-FULL BODY
GO	- COW
SIRAS	- HEAD

KAPALAM	-SKULL
KUKUTAM	-ROOSTER
BAKA	-CROW
UTTANA	- SUPERFICIAL
GAMBIRAM	- DEEP
BADHA	-BOUND
NAUKA	- BOAT
VRIKSHAM	- TREE
VASISTAR	-ANCIENT SAGES
SAMHITHA	-ANCIENT TEXT
SIMHA	-LION
MAYURA	-PEACOCK
NARASIMHA	-JOIN OF MAN AND LION ,THE INCARNATION TAKEN BY LORD VISHNU.
HINDHU	-RELEGION FOLLOWED IN INDIA.
ARDHA	- HALF
PADMA	- LOTUS
NATANAM	- DANCE
VYAYAMA	- EXCERCISE
DIPIKA	- LIGHT
CHATHUR	- FOUR
ANGA	- LIMP, PARTS,
SVA	-DOG

GARUDA	-EAGLE
SETHU	-BRIDGE
BANDHA	-JOINT
HALA	-PLOUGH
CHAKRAM	-WHEEL
NIDRA	-SLEEP
VRICHIKA	-SCORPION
JANU	-KNEE
SWASTHIKA	-AUSPICIOUS
SIDHI	-DIVINE POWER
AMIRTHAM	-NECTOR
VIPARITHA	-REVERSE
SUKHAM	-HAPPY
UPANISAD	-ANCIENT LITERATURE
ADHO	-DOWNWARD
MUKHA	-FACE
TRI	-THREE
MUKTHA	-SALVATION
VIKRAMA	-DIRECTION
DHURUVASAR	-ANCIENT SAGES
BHAIRAVA SIVA	-AN INCARNATION TAKEN BY LORD
KAALAM	-TIME

ANKURAM	-ELEPHANT GOUD
GARBA	-FOETUS
KURMA	-TORTOISE
VIRA	-WARRIOR

------/-------